STEREO ATLAS
OF GLAUCOMA

STEREO ATLAS
OF GLAUCOMA

David G. Campbell, M.D.
Professor of Surgery (Ophthalmology)
Dartmouth Medical School
Hanover, New Hampshire
Director of Glaucoma Service
Dartmouth Hitchcock Medical Center
Lebanon, New Hampshire

Peter A. Netland, M.D., Ph.D.
Associate Professor
Director of Glaucoma
Department of Ophthalmology
University of Tennessee, Memphis
Memphis, Tennessee

with 267 stereo photographs

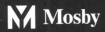

Mosby

St. Louis Baltimore Boston Carlsbad Chicago Minneapolis New York Philadelphia Portland
London Milan Sydney Tokyo Toronto

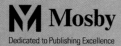

Mosby

Dedicated to Publishing Excellence

A Times Mirror
Company

Senior Editor: Laurel Craven
Developmental Editor: Wendy Buckwalter
Project Manager: Chris Baumle
Production Editor: Marian Hall
Designer: Nancy McDonald
Manufacturing Manager: William A. Winneberger, Jr.

Printed in the United States of America
Composition by Color Associates, Inc.
Lithography/color film by Color Associates, Inc.
Printing/binding by Walsworth Publishing Co.

Mosby-Year Book, Inc.
11830 Westline Industrial Drive
St. Louis, Missouri 63146

Campbell, David G., M.D.
    Stereo atlas of glaucoma / David G. Campbell, Peter A. Netland.—1st ed.
        p.   cm.
    Includes bibliographical references and index.
    ISBN 0-8151-1399-4
    1. Glaucoma—Atlases.   I. Netland, Peter A.   II. Title.
    [DNLM: 1. Glaucoma—atlases.   WW 17 C187s 1998]
RE871.C35   1998
617.7'41'00222—DC21
DNLM/DLC
for Library of Congress   97-22257
                                                               CIP

98 99 00 01 02/9 8 7 6 5 4 3 2 1

To our families, friends, colleagues, and trainees

The idea for this book was sparked by our interactions with trainees in ophthalmology, both at the Lancaster Course in Waterville, Maine, and at our home institutions. As is so often the case, in teaching we learned about the needs of the students and came to a new appreciation of the teaching material itself. It became clear to us that stereo photographs provide a unique and dramatic format for the visual information we use in the diagnosis and management of glaucoma patients. These photographs promote a sudden awareness and lightning bolt-like understanding of information that is difficult or impossible to obtain from written descriptions or two-dimensional images.

We have attempted to simplify the text and to include only essential references. Often the references are to other reviews or textbooks. Whenever possible, we have directed the reader to detailed material in other Mosby publications, including *The Glaucomas*, edited by Robert Ritch, M. Bruce Shields, and Theodore Krupin, and *Becker-Shaffer's Diagnosis and Therapy of the Glaucomas*, edited by H. Dunbar Hoskins Jr. and Michael A. Kass. Several other excellent textbooks of glaucoma exist, providing exhaustive reviews of many of the topics described in this book.

This book is intended for trainees in ophthalmology, particularly those interested in glaucoma, and practitioners who have clinical contact with glaucoma patients. We hope that primary care practitioners who examine the optic nerve will find value in the images contained in this book. In our view, the three-dimensional information in stereo photographs is breathtaking and inspirational, and we hope others will appreciate the beauty and usefulness of this approach.

David G. Campbell, M.D.
Peter A. Netland, M.D., Ph.D.

We are indebted to our mentors, colleagues and patients, who have shaped this book in many ways. In particular, David D. Donaldson, M.D., developed the camera used for many of the images in the book. Photographs for the book were not only from our own collections, but also from those of Dr. Donaldson in the archives at the Massachusetts Eye and Ear Infirmary. We are especially thankful for the expert assistance of Paula C. Reynolds, Deborah A. Vivolo, and Merry B. Post. We are also grateful to Audrey C. Melanson, who contributed her expert photographic and technical assistance. Mosby-Year Book, Inc. provided excellent publishing support through the efforts of Senior Editor Laurel Craven, Developmental Editor Wendy Buckwalter, and Production Editor Marian Hall. For contributing to the Suggested Readings reference lists in Part I, we are greatly appreciative of Robert M. Schertzer, M.D., F.R.C.S.C., Clinical Assistant Professor, Glaucoma, Anterior Segment Surgery & Ophthalmic Informatics, WK Kellogg Eye Center, Ann Arbor, Michigan.

The purpose of this atlas is to present photographs of various glaucomas in a three-dimensional format. This format allows for rapid understanding of the information used in the diagnosis and management of glaucoma patients.

This atlas complements the second edition of *The Glaucomas*, edited by Robert Ritch, Bruce Shields, and Theodore Krupin, as well as other glaucoma publications by Mosby. The textual portion of the atlas is not meant to be exhaustive, and the reader is referred to our other titles for more detailed information on the topics covered in this atlas.

Related titles include Hoskins HD Jr, Kass MA: *Becker-Shaffer's Diagnosis and Therapy of the Glaucomas*, 6th edition; Thomas JV, Belcher CD III, Simmons RD: *Glaucoma Surgery*; Alward WLM: *Color Atlas of Gonioscopy*; Hodapp E, Parris RK II, Anderson DR: *Clinical Decisions in Glaucoma*; Anderson DR: *Automated Static Perimetry*; and Harrington DO, Drake MV: *The Visual Fields: Text and Atlas of Clinical Perimetry*, 6th edition.

The stereo glasses inside the cover of this atlas aid the reader in viewing the images in stereo. Specific instructions for assembling the glasses and viewing the images are printed on the glasses. Replacement viewers may be obtained by calling Mosby customer service at 1-800-633-6699. The images may also be viewed with any +7 diopter lenses.

PART I: THE ANTERIOR SEGMENT   1

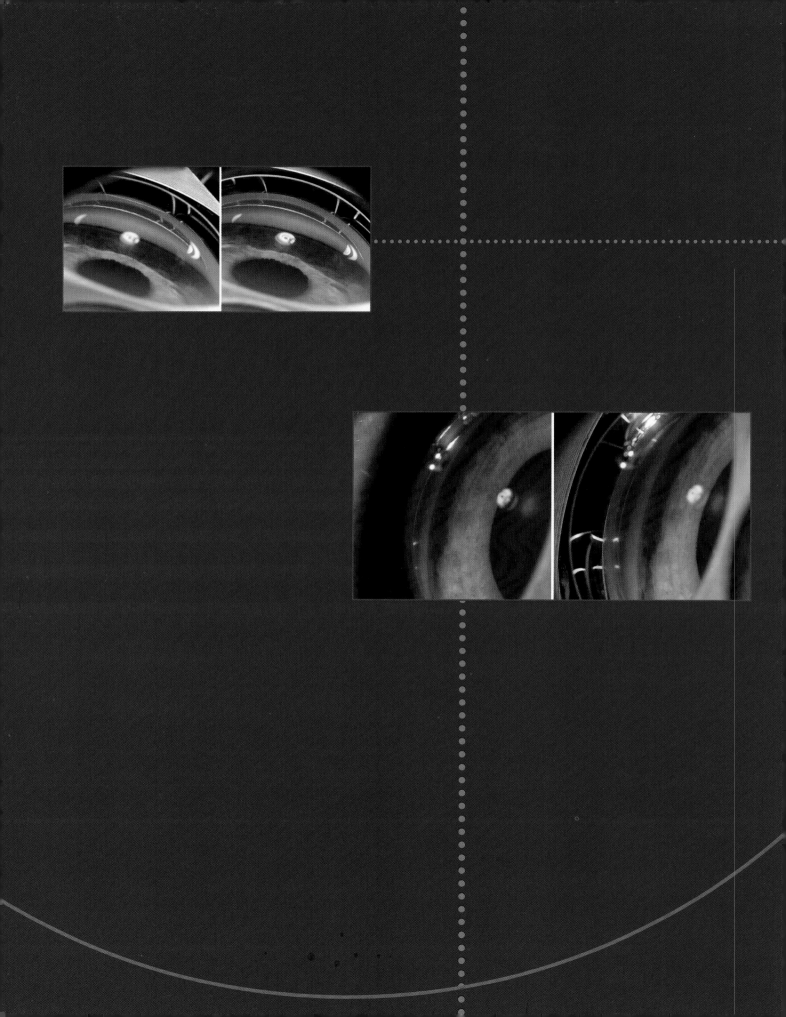

PART ONE

THE ANTERIOR SEGMENT

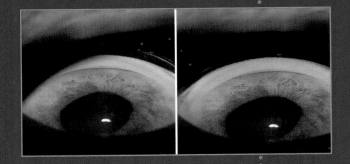

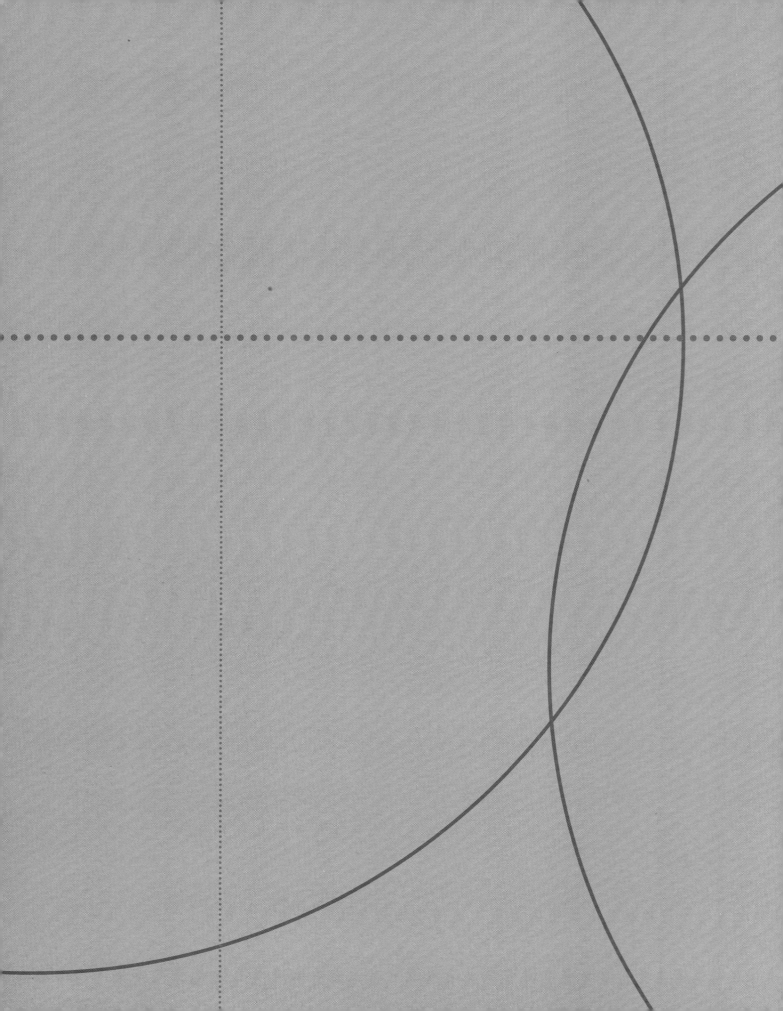

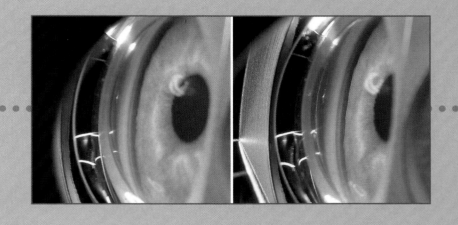

CHAPTER 1

THE NORMAL ANTERIOR
SEGMENT

In the examination of the anterior segment for signs of glaucoma, there are many pathologic findings that will be demonstrated throughout the text. The sclera, the cornea, the anterior chamber, the iris, and the lens should be examined systematically at the slit lamp.

In this chapter, photographs of the normal anterior segment show the normal iris, the normal angle, the greater arterial circle of the iris, the eye in full dilation with a solitary iris process, blood in Schlemm's canal, an injection specimen of Schlemm's canal, and a posterior view of the lens and the ciliary processes.

SUGGESTED READINGS

Alward WLM: Color atlas of gonioscopy, London, England, 1994, Wolfe Publishing (Mosby-Year Book Europe Limited), pp 9–14, 39–49.

Caprioli J: The ciliary epithelia and aqueous humor. In Hart WM Jr, editor: Adler's physiology of the eye, ed 9, St. Louis, 1992, Mosby-Year Book, Inc, pp 228–247.

Grant WM and Schuman JS: The angle of the anterior chamber. In Epstein DL, Allingham RR, and Schuman JS, editors: Chandler and Grant's glaucoma, ed 4, Baltimore, 1997, Williams & Wilkins, pp 51–83.

Hart WM Jr: Intraocular pressure. In Hart WM Jr, editor: Adler's physiology of the eye, ed 9, St. Louis, 1992, Mosby-Year Book, Inc, pp 248–267.

Hoskins HD Jr and Kass MA: Gonioscopic anatomy. In Becker-Shaffer's diagnosis and therapy of the glaucomas, ed 6, St. Louis, 1989, Mosby-Year Book, Inc, pp 101–105.

Tripathi BJ, Tripathi RC, and Wisdom JE: Embryology of the anterior segment of the human eye. In Ritch R, Shields MB, and Krupin T, editors: The glaucomas, ed 2, St. Louis, 1996, Mosby-Year Book, Inc, pp 3–38.

Van Buskirk EM: Anatomy. In Epstein DL, Allingham RR, and Schuman JS, editors: Chandler and Grant's glaucoma, ed 4, Baltimore, 1997, Williams & Wilkins, pp 6–17.

Wiggs JL: Genetics of glaucoma. In Wiggs JL, editor: Molecular genetics of ocular disease, New York, 1994, John Wiley & Sons, Inc, pp 83–98.

Yanoff M and Fine BS: The anterior chamber angle. In Ocular histology, ed 2, Hagerstown, 1979, Harper & Row, pp 251–270.

Fig. 1-1

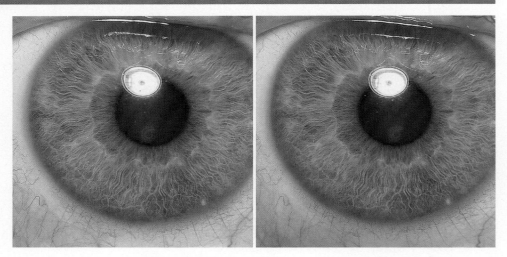

A normal blue iris. Blood-filled radial iris vessels can be seen. Down and to the left, the greater arterial circle of the iris, running much more medial than usual, is visible. The collarette can be seen concentric to the pupil, and between it and the brown, well-formed pupillary ruff, seen through the stroma, is the grayish, circular pupillary sphincter muscle. Yellowish tan, small iris freckles can be seen on the iris surface.

Fig. 1-2

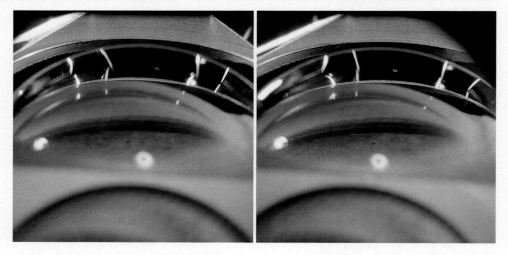

A normal angle. The brown iris recedes into a dark, brown gray ciliary body band. Above this is the white scleral spur, the most prominent landmark in the angle. Above that is the light tan pigmented portion of the trabecular meshwork overlying Schlemm's canal. This portion represents fine, dispersed pigment that has been phagocitized by normal trabecular meshwork endothelial cells. Above this portion of the trabecular meshwork is less pigmented, superior trabecular meshwork tissue, and above this is a wavy, pigmented Schwalbe's line, with flecks of pigment on the trabecular meshwork nearby. This is a Shaffer grade IV, or approximately 40°, wide open angle that is not occludable after dilation.

Fig. 1-3

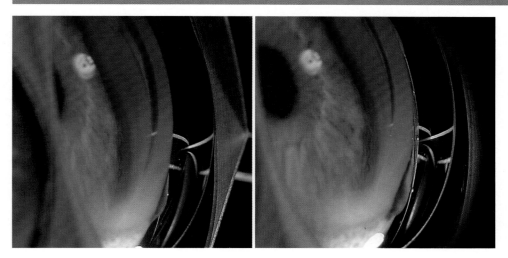

The greater arterial circle of the iris, which can occasionally be seen in the angle as a normal variant, can be seen here.

Fig. 1-4

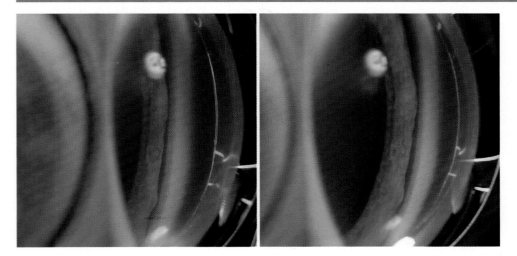

In full dilation this iris may, particularly in younger eyes, lift off the lens, allowing a view of the ciliary processes, as seen here. A solitary iris process can occasionally be seen to insert into the midportion of the trabecular meshwork, which is nonpigmented and translucent in nature and which sits anterior to a gray ciliary body band.

Fig. 1-5

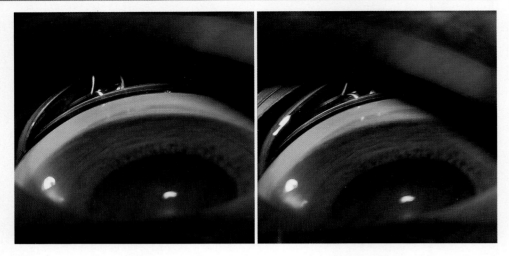

In some eyes, iris processes may be abundant and obscure the scleral spur, as can be seen here where brown iris processes form almost a mat covering the scleral spur. The meshwork is again translucent, and there is no distinct Schwalbe's line.

Fig. 1-6

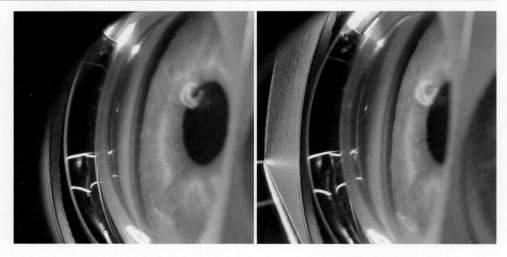

Blood in Schlemm's canal. Occasionally, during gonioscopy, pressure on the limbus will cause a normal reflux of blood into Schlemm's canal. This can help identify the trabecular meshwork. In this blue-eyed patient, Schlemm's canal resides behind the posterior three fifths of the trabecular meshwork, with a normal ciliary band beneath without iris processes. This phenomenon is seen more commonly during supine Koeppe gonioscopy than during upright slit-lamp gonioscopy.

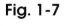

Fig. 1-7

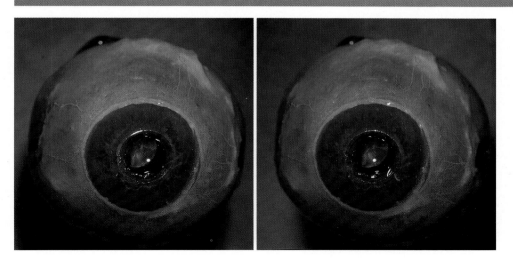

A normal human eye after injection of Schlemm's canal and removal of sclera, showing Schlemm's canal and external collector channels in orange. (Courtesy of Vicente L. Jocson, M.D.)

Fig. 1-8

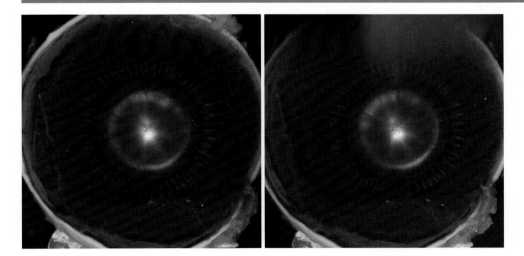

Photograph of normal human eye, dissected, showing the normal ring of ciliary processes surrounding the lens.

Fig. 1-9

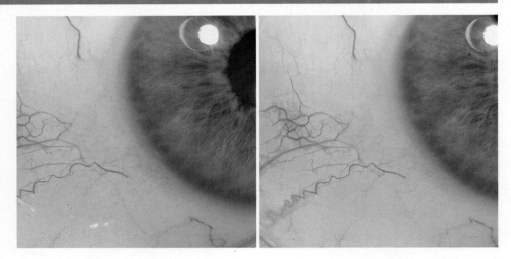

Scleral photograph showing a columnated (or aqueous) vein centrally with a mixture of blood and clear aqueous.

Fig. 1-10

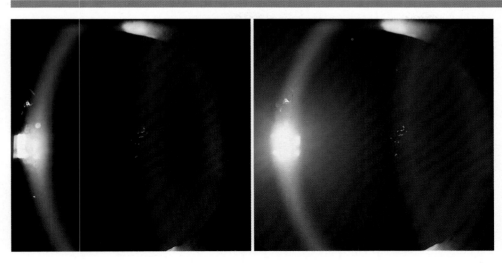

Anterior segment photograph of pigment on the anterior lens surface with stellate or crowsfoot configuration. This type of pigmentation is congenital.

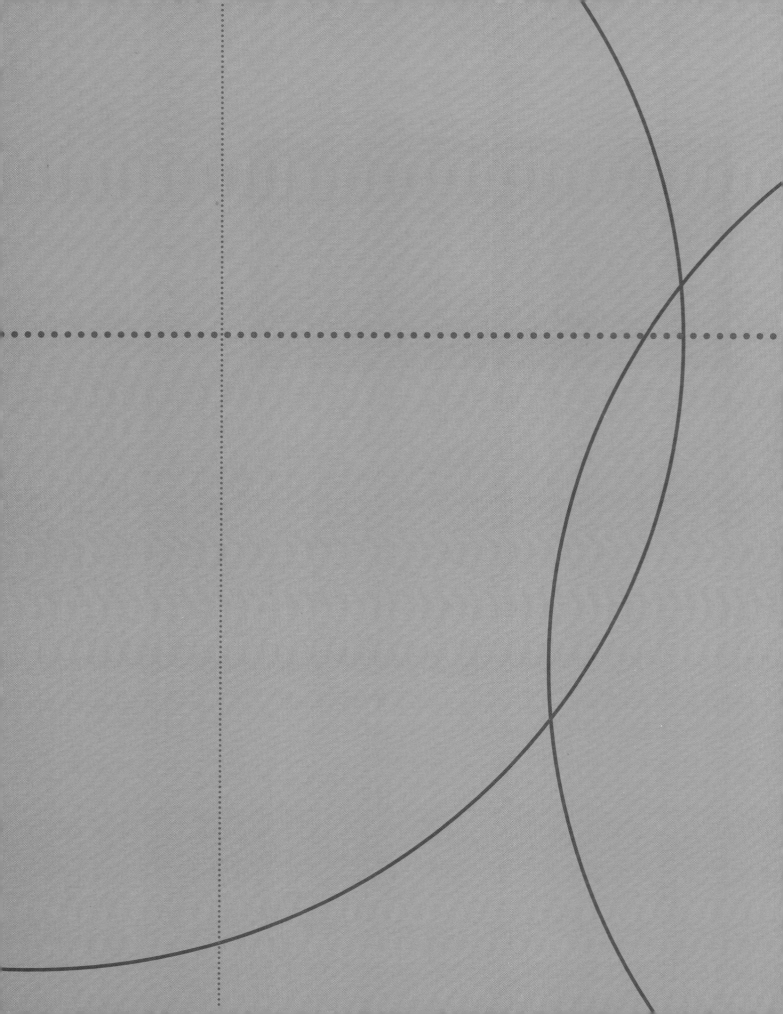

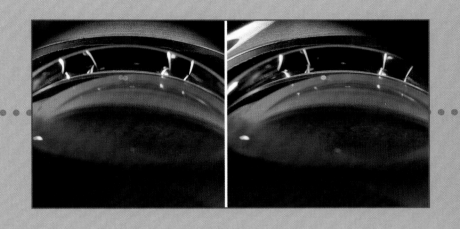

CHAPTER 2

CHRONIC OPEN-ANGLE GLAUCOMA

Chronic open-angle glaucoma is the most common glaucoma seen in the United States and is probably the most common glaucoma seen worldwide. The exact cause of the obstruction to the outflow of aqueous has not been explained fully, and there are a number of different theories as to what may be happening within the trabecular meshwork and/or the outflow channels.

Chronic open-angle glaucoma is generally symmetric. This suggests that the pathologic process within the outflow channels of the eye is also rather symmetric. This can be contrasted with exfoliation glaucoma, for instance, another open-angle glaucoma, which tends to be far more asymmetric.

Gonioscopically, there are no distinguishing features to the appearance of the trabecular meshwork. The diagnosis of chronic open-angle glaucoma is made typically by finding a chronically elevated intraocular pressure, usually in both eyes, without finding evidence of any of the secondary glaucomas. The angle is open, not closed, and generally appears normal.

A finding that can be called segmentation of pigmentation may be observed in eyes with chronic open-angle glaucoma, perhaps more often than in eyes without glaucoma (Fig. 2-1). This segmentation can be seen in eyes that have dispersed a moderate amount of pigment due to normal aging. The pattern cannot be discerned if there has been no dispersal of pigment, which functions as a natural tracer. The darker segments of pigment may indicate regions of preferential flow.

SUGGESTED READINGS

Alvarado JA, Murphy C, and Juster R: Trabecular meshwork cellularity in primary open-angle glaucoma and nonglaucomatous normals. Ophthalmology 91:564, 1984.

Alvarado JA, Yun AJ, and Murphy CG: Juxtacanalicular tissue in primary open-angle glaucoma and in nonglaucomatous normals. Arch Ophthalmol 104:1517, 1986.

American Academy of Ophthalmology Preferred Practice Patterns Committee, Glaucoma Panel: Primary open-angle glaucoma suspect, San Francisco, 1995, American Academy of Ophthalmology.

Epstein DL: Primary open angle glaucoma. In Epstein DL, Allingham RR, and Schuman JS, editors: Chandler and Grant's glaucoma, ed 4, Baltimore, 1997, Williams & Wilkins, pp 183–198.

Hoskins HD Jr and Kass MA: Primary open-angle glaucoma. In Becker-Shaffer's diagnosis and therapy of the glaucomas, ed 6, St. Louis, 1989, Mosby-Year Book, Inc, pp 277–307.

Kahn HA et al: The Framingham Eye Study: I. Outline and major prevalence findings. Am J Epidemiol 106:17, 1977.

Klein BEK et al: Prevalence of glaucoma: the Beaver Dam Eye Study. Ophthalmology 99:1499, 1992.

Migdal C, Gregory W, and Hitchings R: Long-term functional outcome after early surgery compared with laser and medicine in open-angle glaucoma. Ophthalmology 101:1651, 1994.

Sommer A et al: Relationship between intraocular pressure and primary open angle glaucoma among white and black Americans: the Baltimore Eye Survey. Arch Ophthalmol 109: 1090, 1991.

Tielsch JM et al: Racial variations in the prevalence of primary open-angle glaucoma: the Baltimore Eye Survey. JAMA 226:369, 1991.

Wilson MR and Martone JF: Epidemiology of chronic open-angle glaucoma. In Ritch R, Shields MB, and Krupin T, editors: The glaucomas, ed 2, St. Louis, 1996, Mosby-Year Book, Inc, pp 753–768.

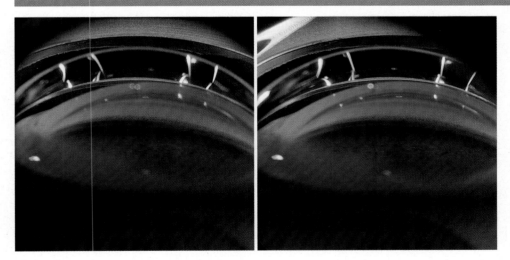

Fig. 2-1

The inferior angle of a patient with chronic open-angle glaucoma. There are no diagnostic features on gonioscopy that can definitely identify a patient with chronic open-angle glaucoma from normal. Note segments of heavier pigmentation adjacent to segments of lighter pigmentation.

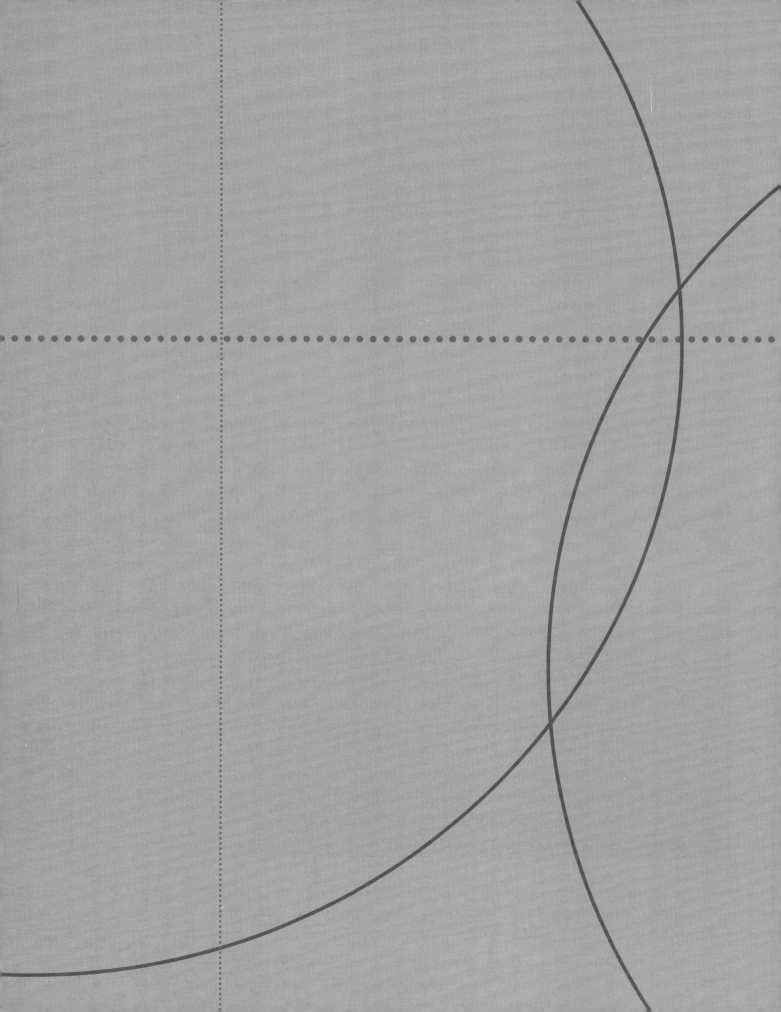

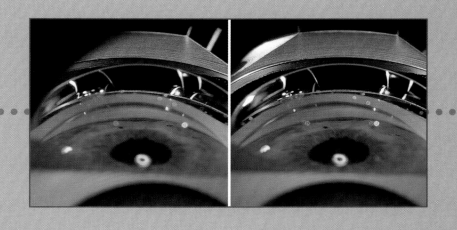

CHAPTER 3

THE ANGLE-CLOSURE GLAUCOMAS

The angle-closure glaucomas comprise a group of diseases in which the angle becomes closed and the trabecular meshwork becomes covered by the peripheral iris, either appositionally or synechially.

When forces anterior to the iris pull the iris onto the trabecular meshwork, the closure is synechial (i.e., neovascular glaucoma, essential iris atrophy, inflammatory contact due to keratic precipitates, etc.). When forces posterior to the iris push the peripheral iris forward, a group of primary and secondary angle-closure glaucomas result.

The most common type of primary angle-closure glaucoma in the United States is relative pupillary block angle-closure glaucoma. Here, in general, the combination of a small eye, combined with increasing lens size and increasing miosis with aging, leads to increased central irido-lenticular apposition. This creates a slightly higher pressure in the posterior chamber than in the anterior, causing the peripheral iris to bulge forward slightly. This forward movement of the peripheral iris, in an eye with a narrow angle, can lead to closure, either acute or chronic.

If, in this situation, the iris dilates slightly (in response to darkness or emotional distress), the peripheral iris may become more relaxed, allowing it to bulge even further forward and causing complete and sudden closure, which is the acute angle-closure glaucoma attack.

In a second type of primary angle-closure glaucoma, plateau iris configuration angle-closure glaucoma, relative pupillary block plays less of a role. Forward rotation of the ciliary processes may push the peripheral iris forward, closing the angle.

In a rarer type of angle-closure glaucoma, the lens moves abnormally far forward for an unknown reason, closing the angle.

Lens enlargement, as with a hypermature lens, can cause angle-closure.

A few of the many angle-closure glaucomas are shown in the photographs. Indention gonioscopy and the chamber-deepening procedure also are illustrated.

SUGGESTED READINGS

Alward WLM: Color atlas of gonioscopy, London, England, 1994, Wolfe Publishing (Mosby-Year Book Europe Limited), pp 67–86.

Campbell DG and Vela A: Modern goniosynechialysis for the treatment of synechial angle-closure glaucoma. Ophthalmology 91: 1052, 1984.

Campbell DG: Primary angle-closure glaucoma. In Albert DA and Jakobiec FA, editors: Principles and practice of ophthalmology, Philadelphia, 1994, WB Saunders Co, pp 1365–1388.

Chandler PA and Simmons RJ: Anterior chamber deepening for gonioscopy at time of surgery. Arch Ophthalmol 74:177, 1965.

Epstein DL: Angle-closure glaucomas. In Epstein DL, Allingham RR and Schuman JS, editors: Chandler and Grant's glaucoma, ed 4, Baltimore, 1997, Williams & Wilkins, pp 235–280.

Epstein DL: Angle-closure glaucoma due to multiple cysts of the iris and ciliary body. In Epstein DL, Allingham RR, and Schuman JS, editors: Chandler and Grant's glaucoma, ed 4, Baltimore, 1997, Williams & Wilkins, pp 334–336.

Forbes M: Gonioscopy with corneal indentation. Arch Ophthalmol 76:488, 1966.

Hoskins HD Jr and Kass MA: Angle-closure glaucoma with pupillary block and angle-closure glaucoma without pupillary block. In Becker-Shaffer's diagnosis and therapy of the glaucomas, ed 6, St. Louis, 1989, Mosby-Year Book, Inc, pp 208–276.

Jin JC and Anderson DR: Laser and unsutured sclerectomy in nanophthalmos. Am J Ophthalmol 109:575, 1990.

Levene R: A new concept of malignant glaucoma. Arch Ophthalmol 87:497, 1972.

Pavlin CJ, Ritch R, and Foster FS: Ultrasound biomicroscopy in plateau iris syndrome. Am J Ophthalmol 113:390, 1992.

Ritch R and Lowe RF: Angle-closure glaucoma: mechanisms and epidemiology and clinical types. In Ritch R, Shields MB, and Krupin T, editors: The glaucomas, ed 2, St. Louis, 1996, Mosby-Year Book, Inc, pp 801–840.

Simmons RJ and Simmons RB: Nanophthalmos: diagnosis and treatment. In Epstein DL, Allingham RR, and Schuman JS, editors: Chandler and Grant's glaucoma, ed 4, Baltimore, 1997, Williams & Wilkins, pp 304–308.

Vela A, Rieser JC, and Campbell DG: The heredity and treatment of angle-closure glaucoma secondary to iris and ciliary body cysts. Ophthalmology 91:332, 1984.

Wand M et al: Plateau iris syndrome. Trans Am Acad Ophthalmol Otolaryngol 83:122, 1977.

Fig. 3-1

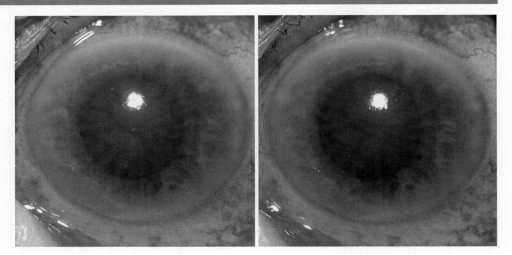

Anterior segment photograph of acute angle-closure glaucoma. The cornea is edematous; the anterior chamber is shallow; the intraocular pressure is high; and the pupil is fixed in mid-dilation, generally 4–5 mm.

Fig. 3-2

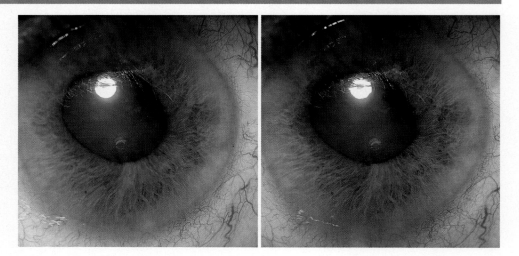

Anterior segment photograph of patient after an attack of acute angle-closure glaucoma. The pupil is fixed and paralyzed in mid-dilation, there are areas of grayish iris atrophy surrounding the sphincter and to the right, and there are small white patches in the anterior lens (glaucomflecken).

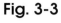

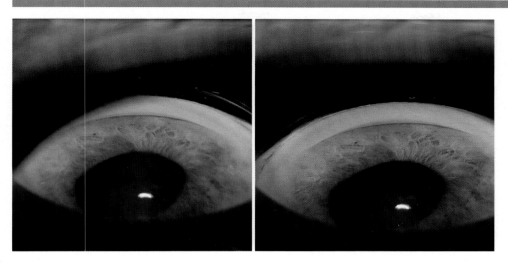

Goniophotograph of the same patient as shown in Fig. 3-2. The angle remains entirely closed with no trabecular meshwork visible. One does not know at this point whether the closure is appositional or synechial.

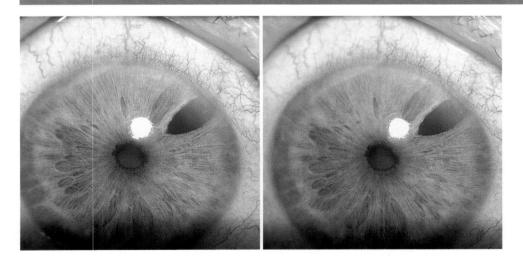

Anterior segment photograph of a patient with relative pupillary block angle-closure glaucoma who has had an incomplete surgical iridectomy in an effort to relieve the block. See Fig. 3-5 for more details.

Fig. 3-5

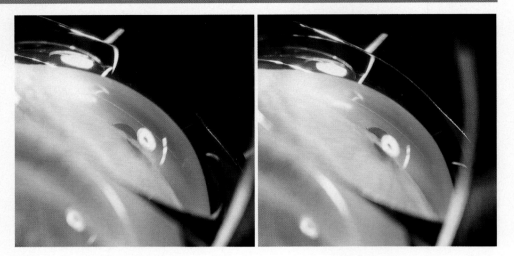

Goniophotograph of the same patient as Fig. 3-4 with relative pupillary block angle-closure glaucoma who has had an incomplete surgical iridectomy in an effort to relieve the block. The stroma of the iris was removed but not the impermeable posterior pigmented layer, which, on gonioscopy, can be seen to bulge into the anterior chamber, indicating the pressure is greater in the posterior chamber than it is in the anterior chamber.

Fig. 3-6

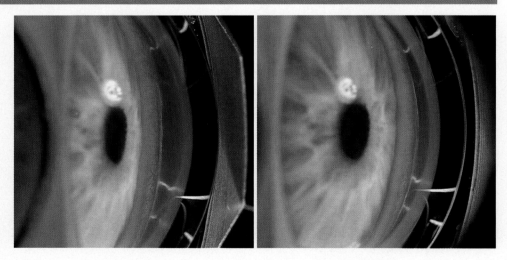

Moderate to marked iris convexity and an apparently narrow or closed angle. This is an example of an insufficient view: The examiner needs to see the depth of the angle to make an accurate assessment, and must change the angle of the view to do so.

Fig. 3-7

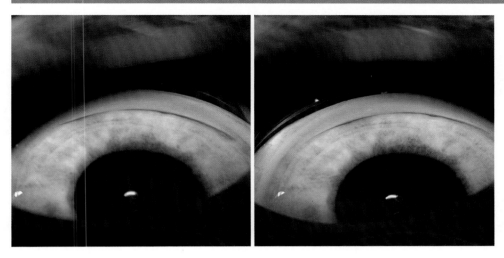

Much angle-closure after mid-dilation of the pupil. The view over the convex iris is sufficient, and the angle is visible. The trabecular meshwork is covered completely on each side laterally and for one clock hour straight ahead. Elsewhere, the anterior trabecular meshwork can be glimpsed.

Fig. 3-8

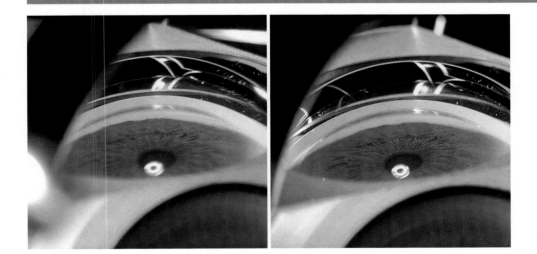

Chronic angle-closure glaucoma. There is moderate iris convexity and complete closure straight ahead for approximately two clock hours. To the right, the angle is narrow but completely open, and to the left, the anterior half of the trabecular meshwork is visible.

Fig. 3-9

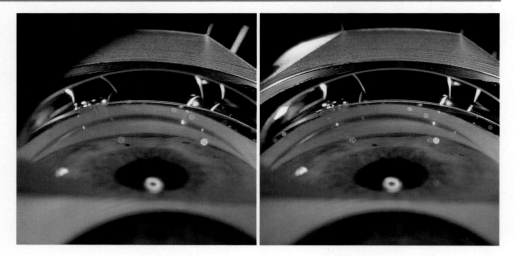

Chronic angle-closure glaucoma with mild iris convexity but with an angle that is almost completely closed. Straight ahead, approximately three-fourths of the trabecular meshwork can be seen for approximately one clock hour. The scleral spur is not seen. Tiny portions of the anterior meshwork can be seen in some other places.

Fig. 3-10

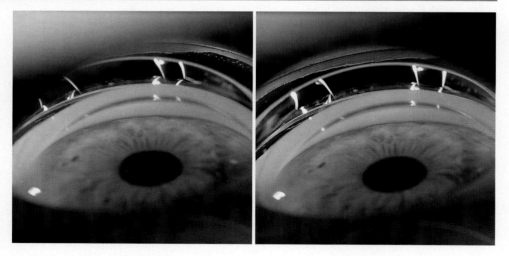

Chronic angle-closure glaucoma with moderate iris convexity and a closed angle. Only the barest portions of the anterior trabecular meshwork, non-pigmented, can be seen.

Fig. 3-11

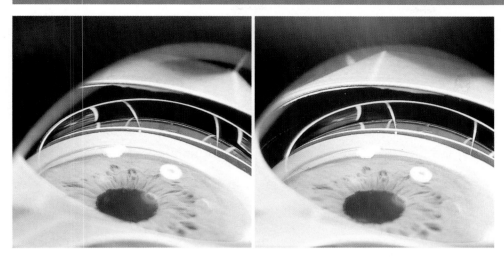

Indentation gonioscopy. Goniophotograph of a patient with angle-closure showing a closed angle on the right. On the left, only the anterior trabecular meshwork is visible. The view was obtained by a noncontact, three-mirror gonioscopy lens.

Fig. 3-12

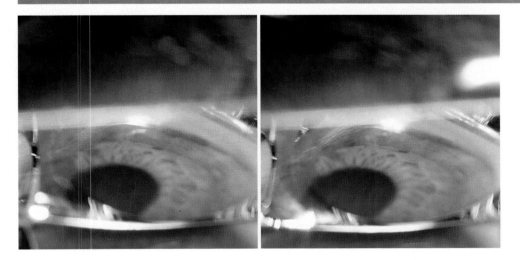

Indentation gonioscopy. The same patient in Fig. 3-11 after indentation gonioscopy with a contact, four-mirror gonioscopy lens. The peripheral iris has been flattened by the indentation, and the angle is entirely open, indicating that the closure was appositional and not synechial.

Fig. 3-13

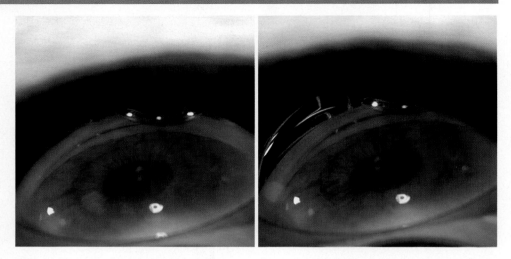

The chamber-deepening procedure. Marked iris convexity and complete angle-closure. The trabecular meshwork is not visible anywhere.

Fig. 3-14

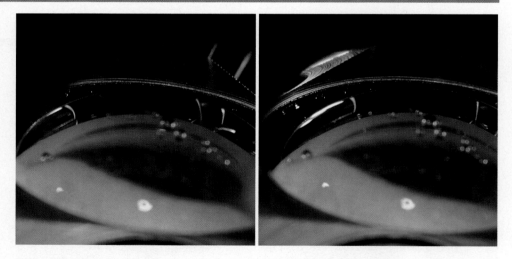

The chamber-deepening procedure. A goniophotograph of the same patient after surgical chamber deepening. A paracentesis has been made and the chamber artificially deepened with fluid. This has dilated the pupil and pressed the peripheral iris posteriorly, revealing that most of the angle-closure was appositional, because the scleral spur now can be seen to the left. Straight ahead there is peripheral anterior synechia formation for one clock hour, covering the scleral spur. The appropriate surgical procedure now can be chosen, if necessary. This deepened configuration allows safe angle surgery, such as goniosynechialysis.

Fig. 3-15

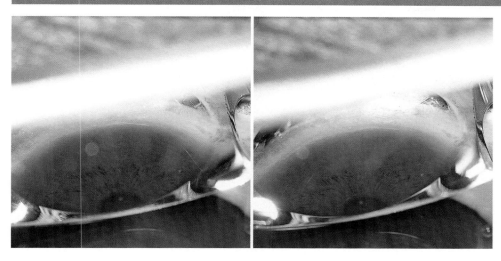

Indentation goniophotograph of same patient with chronic angle-closure glaucoma shown in Fig. 3-8. In the portion of the angle shown, the midportion of the iris is depressed and slightly concave at the edge of the lens, but the peripheral iris elevates to a synechially and completely closed angle in this region. The trabecular meshwork is covered and not visible.

Fig. 3-16

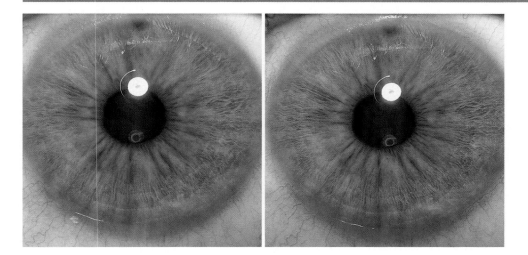

Plateau iris angle-closure. Anterior segment photograph of a patient who has had a surgical iridectomy for angle-closure glaucoma but who continues to have attacks of angle-closure glaucoma. The central chamber is relatively deep in contrast to the shallow chamber of the patient with relative pupillary block angle-closure glaucoma.

Fig. 3-17

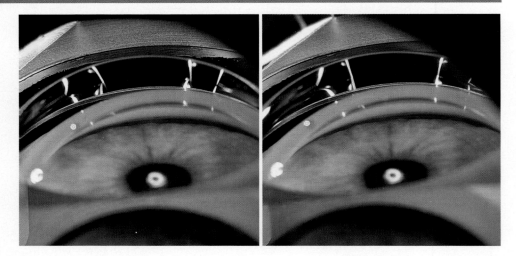

Plateau iris angle-closure. Goniophotograph of same patient as in Fig. 3-16 showing a relatively flat iris and a fall off at the periphery, like the edge of a plateau, into a narrow angle. This angle was capable of closure with dilation despite the presence of a peripheral iridectomy and relief of relative pupillary block.

Fig. 3-18

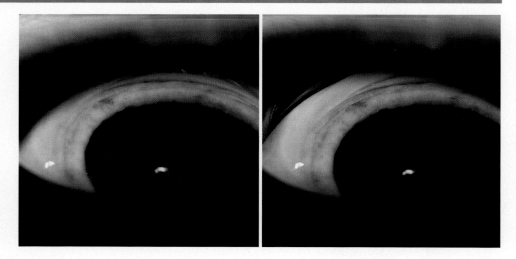

A goniophotograph of a patient with plateau iris configuration angle-closure following pharmacologic dilation. The angle is closed to the left and to the right. Straight ahead, only the anterior portion of the trabecular meshwork is seen. The edge of the lens can be faintly seen, indicating that the iris is off the lens surface and that no relative pupillary block exists.

Fig. 3-19

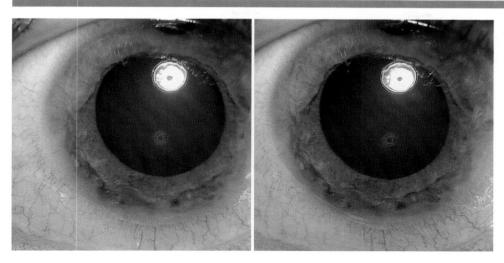

An anterior segment photograph of a patient with mobile lens syndrome angle-closure glaucoma. In this syndrome, the lens can move forward excessively, causing severe angle-closure with unusual high peripheral anterior synechia. The eyes behave as if they had malignant angle-closure glaucoma and respond somewhat to mydriatic cycloplegic therapy, a therapy contraindicated for relative pupillary block and plateau iris angle-closure glaucoma.

Fig. 3-20

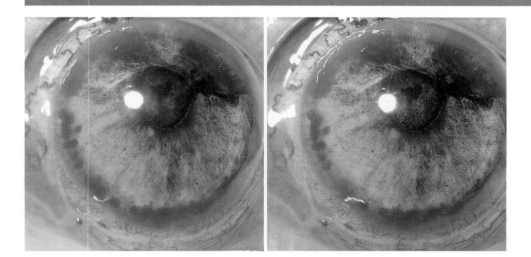

Nanophthalmos. Anterior segment view of a patient with nanophthalmos and severe angle-closure. The eyes are so small that occasionally all attempts to prevent closure fail. This patient has had surgical iridectomy and laser peripheral iridoplasty in an attempt to prevent closure.

Fig. 3-21

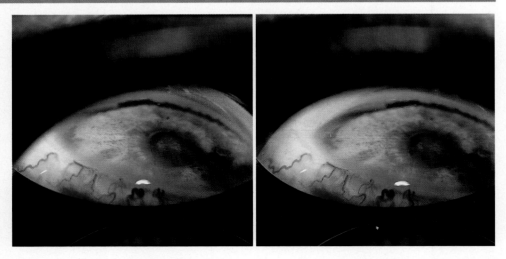

Nanophthalmos. Goniophotograph of same patient in Fig. 3-20 showing that the angle remains open to the left and that the peripheral iris is depressed because of the peripheral iridoplasty but that the angle straight ahead is pigmented and synechially closed.

Fig. 3-22

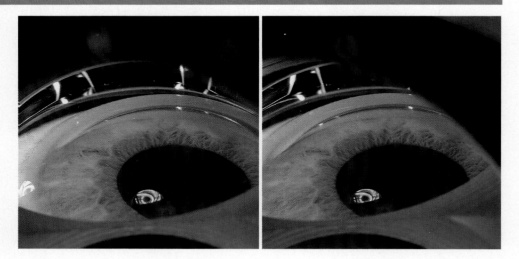

Angle-closure secondary to peripheral iris and ciliary body cysts. Goniophotograph of a patient with large iris cysts originating from the posterior iris surface, seen in the pupillary space, causing complete angle-closure.

Fig. 3-23

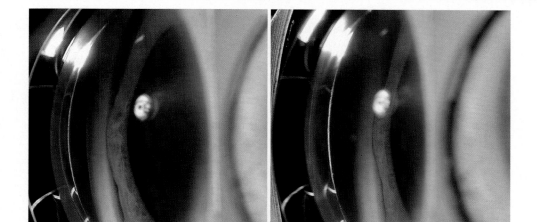

Goniophotograph of a different patient showing centrally a solitary cyst, causing local angle-closure.

Fig. 3-24

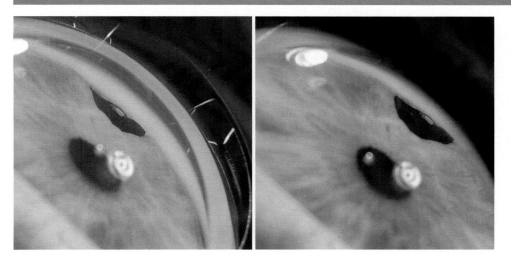

Angle-closure secondary to peripheral iris and ciliary body cysts. Complete angle-closure due to a 360° ring of peripheral iris and ciliary body cysts that are smaller than those seen above. The cysts can be seen through a surgical iridectomy created at the time of filtration surgery. The angle is completely closed synechially.

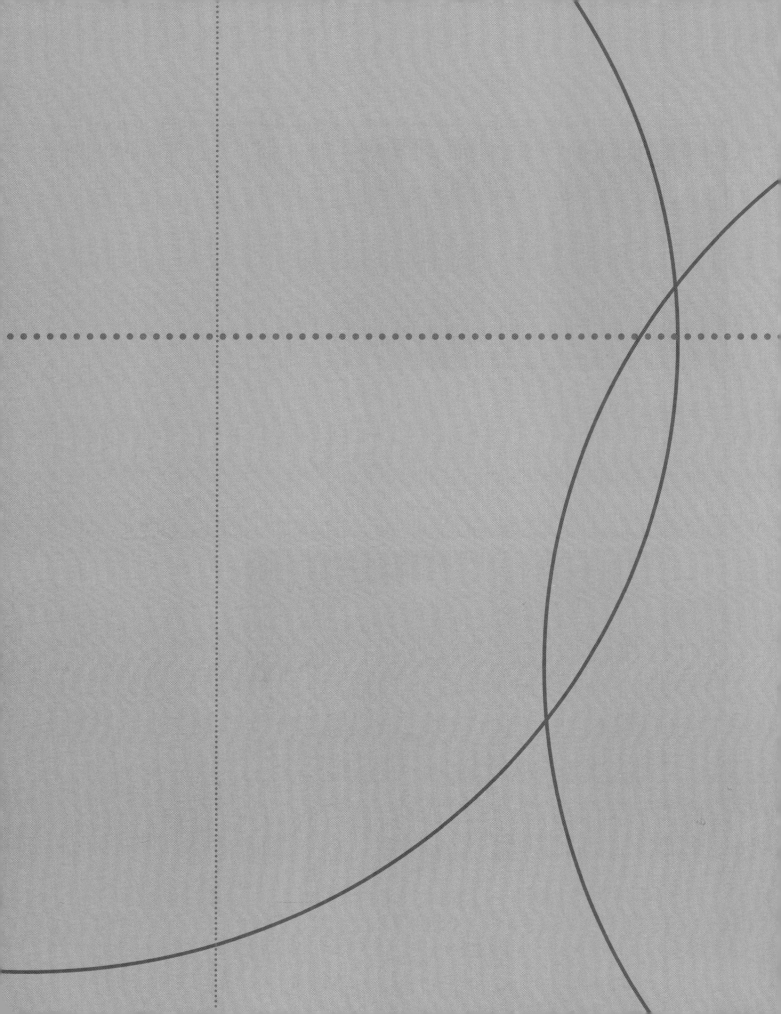

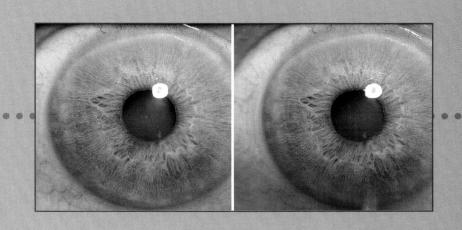

CHAPTER 4

EXFOLIATION GLAUCOMA

Exfoliation glaucoma is a secondary open-angle glaucoma that occurs primarily in the elderly. This glaucoma is associated with the appearance of a fine, gray, dandruff-like material that collects in the posterior and anterior chambers. The material is carried to the trabecular meshwork, where it causes a secondary obstruction and abnormal elevation of intraocular pressure that can then cause glaucomatous damage to the optic nerve. The material often is first seen as fine, gray flecks on the pupillary margin. Dilation of the pupil reveals that the material collects on the anterior surface of the lens. The material then can be rubbed off the surface of the lens by the central iris, leaving a characteristic pattern on the anterior lens surface of a central disc, a surrounding clear zone, and a more peripheral collection of the exfoliation material that fades toward the equator. In the posterior chamber, if there is visual access, the material can be seen on the ciliary processes. The material also can coat the zonules, which can be seen gonioscopically. Pathologic examination reveals that the material coats the posterior surface of the iris. As the material breaks free, it may occasionally adhere to the corneal endothelium. Gonioscopy may reveal flakes of the material deep in the angle and on the surface of the trabecular meshwork. Pathologic sections show that the material is found within the intertrabecular spaces as well.

Occasionally, abnormally heavy amounts of pigment are dispersed within the eye as well, and this pigment can darken the trabecular meshwork. This pigment can highlight Schwalbe's line, particularly inferiorly, and can cause the appearance of fine, undulating lines of pigment, concentric with Schwalbe's line and slightly anterior to it as well.

The figures show exfoliation material at the pupillary margin; the classic appearance of exfoliation material on the anterior surface of the lens; the anterior lens pattern without a central disc; the material rubbed off the anterior surface of the lens in sheet-like fashion; the material on the endothelium; the material deep within the angle; the material coating the ciliary processes; and a finely pigmented trabecular meshwork with an additional line of pigment anterior to the trabecular meshwork (Sampaolesi's line). In this text, we refer to this entity as exfoliation glaucoma, although it is known by other names, including pseudoexfoliation glaucoma.

SUGGESTED READINGS

Alward WLM: Color atlas of gonioscopy, London, England, 1994, Wolfe Publishing (Mosby-Year Book Europe Limited), pp 90–91.

Eagle RC, Font RL, and Fine BS: The basement membrane exfoliation syndrome, Arch Ophthalmol 97:510, 1979.

Epstein DL: Exfoliation and open-angle glaucoma. In Epstein DL, Allingham RR, and Schuman JS, editors: Chandler and Grant's glaucoma, ed 4, Baltimore, 1997, Williams & Wilkins, pp 212–219.

Hoskins HD Jr and Kass MA: Secondary open-angle glaucoma. In Becker-Shaffer's diagnosis and therapy of the glaucomas, ed 6, St. Louis, 1989, Mosby-Year Book, Inc, pp 312–315.

Netland PA et al: Elastosis of the lamina cribrosa in pseudoexfoliation syndrome with glaucoma. Ophthalmology 102:878, 1995.

Richardson TM and Epstein DL: Exfoliation glaucoma: a quantitative perfusion and ultrastructural study. Ophthalmology 88:968, 1981.

Ringvold A and Vegge T: Electron microscopy of the trabecular meshwork in eyes with exfoliation syndrome (pseudoexfoliation of the lens capsule). Virchows Arch (Pathol Anat) 353:110, 1971.

Ringvold A et al: The middle-Norway eye-screening study: II. Prevalence of simple and capsular glaucoma. Acta Ophthalmol 69:273, 1991.

Ritch R: Exfoliation syndrome. In Ritch R, Shields MB, and Krupin T, editors: The glaucomas, ed 2, St. Louis, 1996, Mosby-Year Book, Inc, pp 993–1022.

Fig. 4-1

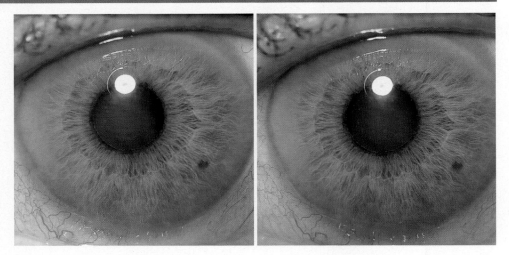

An anterior segment view demonstrating a fine collection of exfoliation material along the pupillary margin in this blue-eyed patient. There is loss of pupillary ruff, also a characteristic of this syndrome.

Fig. 4-2

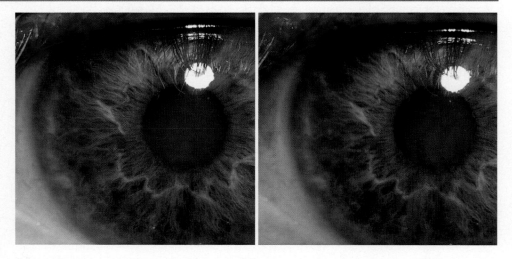

An anterior segment view shows exfoliation material at the pupillary margin, associated with a characteristic loss of the pupillary ruff. At the 11 o'clock position, a piece of the exfoliation material extends into the anterior chamber.

Fig. 4-3

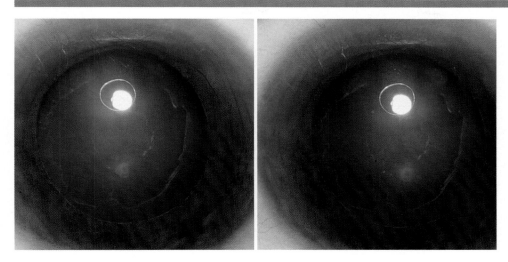

An anterior segment view of the typical exfoliation pattern seen on the anterior surface of the lens after dilation, in a brown-eyed patient. The pattern shows a central disc, a clear zone surrounding this disc, and a peripheral zone of exfoliation material.

Fig. 4-4

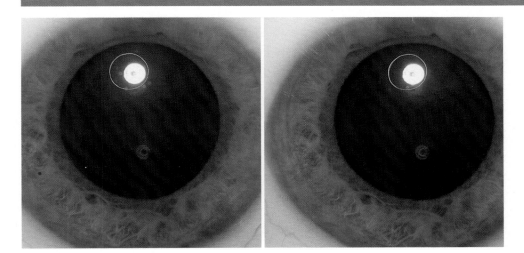

An anterior segment view shows, again, the classic lenticular pattern on the anterior surface of the lens.

Fig. 4-5

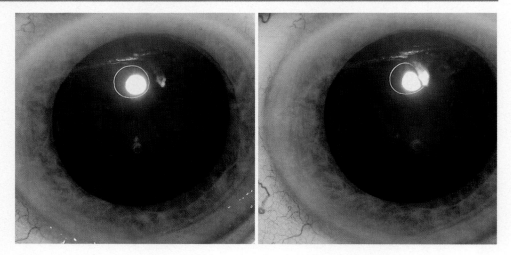

Another anterior segment view of the classic lenticular pattern.

Fig. 4-6

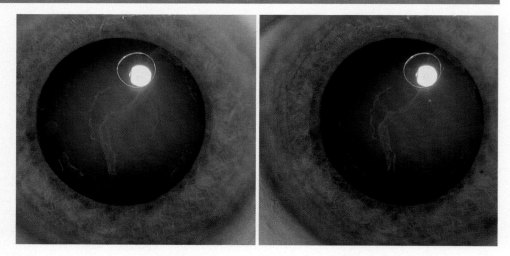

An anterior segment view of the classic lenticular pattern, revealing sheet-like dislocation of the exfoliation material.

Fig. 4-7

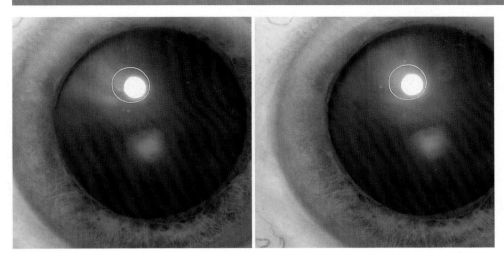

An anterior segment view of the peripheral appearance of exfoliation material on the anterior surface of the lens, showing the absence of a central disc.

Fig. 4-8

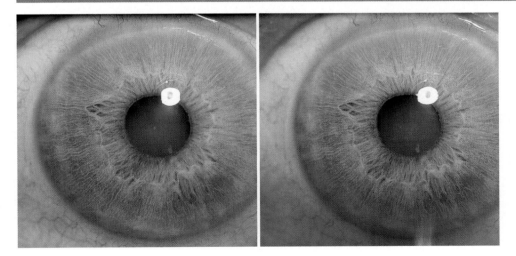

An anterior segment reveals a patient with a shallow anterior chamber, with exfoliation material central on the endothelium, along with the characteristic pattern of exfoliation at the pupillary margin, with loss of the pupillary ruff. A mild amount of pigment dispersion can be seen as fine pigment accumulation on the anterior surface of the iris, particularly around the collarette and the inferior portion of the iris.

Fig. 4-9

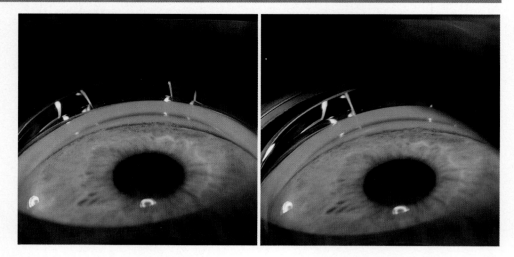

A goniophotograph of the same eye shown in Fig. 4-8. The flecks of exfoliation material can be seen on the endothelium, slightly out of focus. A narrow angle can be seen with rather significant iris convexity, and, in the angle recess, flecks of exfoliation material can be seen.

Fig. 4-10

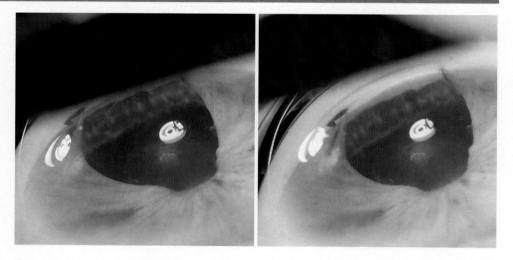

A gonioscopic view of a patient who has had an intracapsular cataract extraction with sector iridectomy. A whitish layer of exfoliation material can be seen coating the surfaces of the ciliary processes. The material tends to collect, not on the anterior surface of the ciliary processes, but more posteriorly. Herniated vitreous, with a partially intact anterior hyaloid face, can be seen at the inferior pupillary margin. Wisps of iris on each side of the sector iridectomy can be seen adhering to the internal edge of the cataract incision.

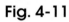

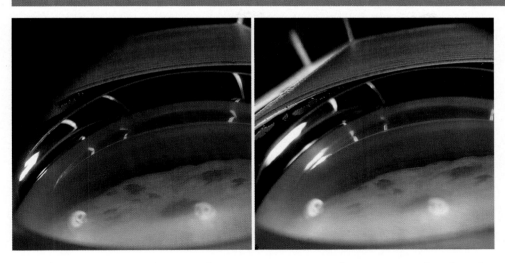

An inferior gonioscopic view showing, anterior to the pigmented trabecular meshwork, a fine, undulating pigment line characteristic of Sampaolesi's line.

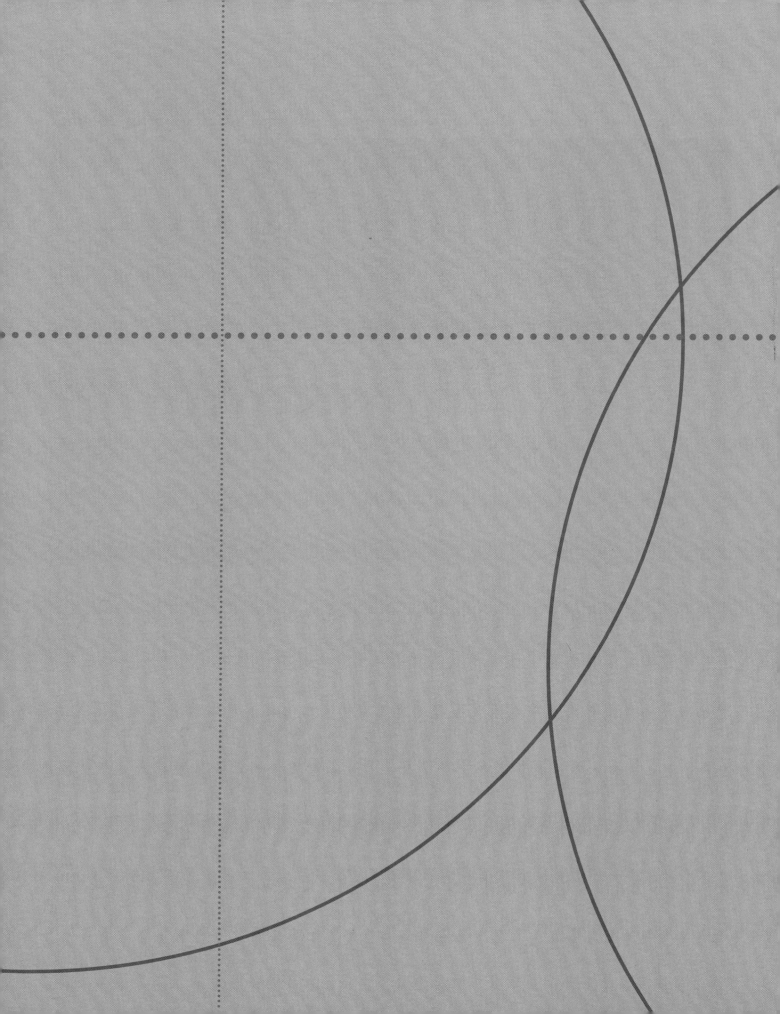

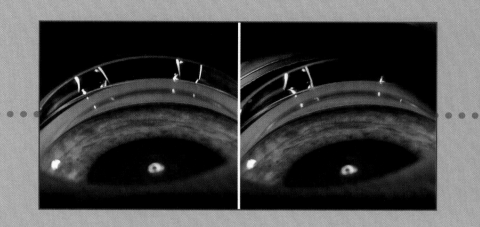

CHAPTER 5

PIGMENTARY GLAUCOMA

Pigmentary glaucoma is an uncommon open-angle glaucoma that is associated with an excessive dispersion of pigment within the posterior and anterior chambers. When carried to the trabecular meshwork, this pigment causes obstruction with elevation of intraocular pressure. Recent studies have shown that in this syndrome, the pressure is intermittently higher in the anterior chamber than it is in the posterior chamber. Elevated anterior pressure forces the peripheral iris posteriorly, causing it to rub against packets of zonules that hold the lens in place. This rubbing causes a release of pigment from the posterior surface of the iris, resulting in characteristic, peripheral, radial transillumination defects. The dispersed pigment can be seen in a circular line on the posterior surface of the lens and as free pigment on the anterior surface of the iris. On and within the endothelium, dispersed pigment appears as a Krukenberg spindle. Heavy deposits are visible within the trabecular meshwork itself, where they appear as an even band of pigment for 360°.

Photographs of a Krukenberg spindle, iris transillumination defects, characteristic peripheral iris concavity, and heavy pigmentation within the trabecular meshwork itself illustrate this condition. A flattening of the posterior iris concavity is shown that was caused by relieving the inverse pupillary block peculiar to this syndrome. The final figure in this series shows the angle of a patient in whom secondary pigmentary glaucoma developed due to chafing by an intraocular lens.

SUGGESTED READINGS

Campbell DG: Pigmentary dispersion and glaucoma: a new theory. Arch Ophthalmol 97:1667, 1979.

Campbell DG and Schertzer RM: Pigmentary glaucoma. In Ritch R, Shields MB, and Krupin T, editors: The glaucomas, ed 2, St. Louis, 1996, Mosby-Year Book, Inc, pp 975–991.

Epstein DL: Pigment dispersion and pigmentary glaucoma. In Epstein DL, Allingham RR, and Schuman JS, editors: Chandler and Grant's glaucoma, ed 4, Baltimore, 1997, Williams & Wilkins, pp 220–231.

Karickhoff JR: Pigment dispersion syndrome and pigmentary glaucoma: a new mechanism concept, a new treatment, and a new technique. Ophthalmic Surg 23:269, 1992.

Liebmann JM et al: Prevention of blinking alters iris configuration in pigment dispersion syndrome and in normal eyes. Ophthalmology 102:446, 1995.

Pavlin CJ, Harasiewicz K, and Foster FS: Posterior iris bowing in pigmentary dispersion syndrome caused by accommodation. Am J Ophthalmol 118:390, 1994.

Pavlin CJ et al: Ultrasound biomicroscopic features of pigmentary glaucoma. Can J Ophthalmol 29:187, 1994.

Pavlin CJ et al: Accommodation and iridotomy in the pigment dispersion syndrome. Ophthalmic Surg Lasers 27:113, 1996.

Richardson TM, Hutchinson BT, and Grant WM: The outflow tract in pigmentary glaucoma: a light and electron microscopic study. Arch Ophthalmol 95:1015, 1977.

Sokol J et al: Location of the iris insertion in pigment dispersion syndrome. Ophthalmology 103:289, 1996.

Sugar HS: Pigmentary glaucoma: a 24 year review. Am J Ophthalmol 2:499, 1966.

Sugar HS and Barbour FA: Pigmentary glaucoma: a rare clinical entity. Am J Ophthalmol 32:90, 1949.

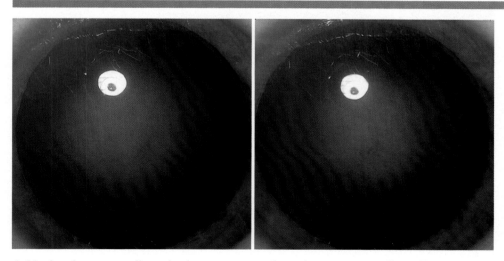

Fig. 5-1

A Krukenberg spindle, which is pigment that characteristically collects on the central corneal endothelium, usually in a vertical pattern. The spindle often is the first sign of pigmentary glaucoma that is seen at slit-lamp examination. When a spindle is seen, other signs of pigmentary dispersion glaucoma should be looked for. Occasionally, the collection of pigment on the surface of the cornea can be quite light, even when there is heavy pigmentation elsewhere.

Fig. 5-2

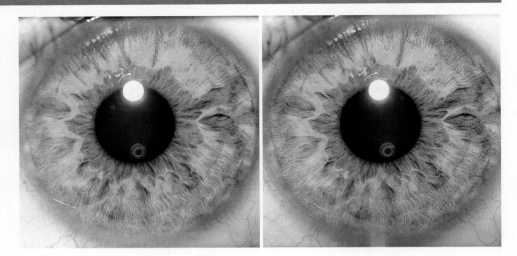

A collection of abnormal pigment on the surface of the iris that can be seen frequently in this syndrome. Very rarely, this pigmentation can be so heavy that it causes a heterochromia.

Fig. 5-3

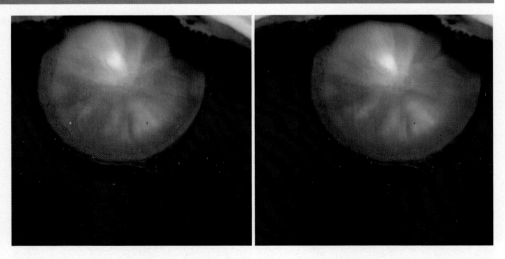

A pathology specimen showing the collection of pigment on the posterior surface of the lens that commonly occurs in this syndrome as pigment collects in the area between the periphery of the lens and the attachment of the hyaloid.

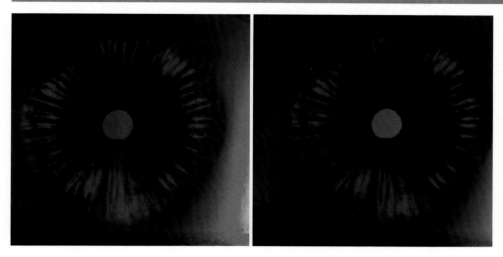

Fig. 5-4

The characteristic, peripheral, radial transillumination defects that are pathognomonic of this syndrome. These defects can increase in number as the syndrome progresses.

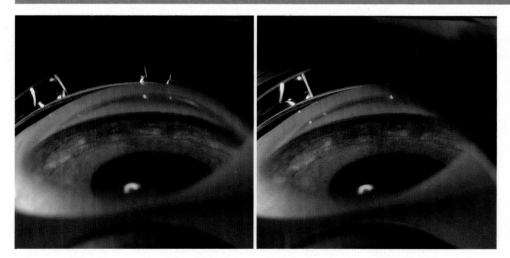

Fig. 5-5

A goniophotograph showing the characteristic peripheral iris concavity that typically is seen in this syndrome. This aberrant configuration of the iris leads to the unusual loss of pigment.

Fig. 5-6

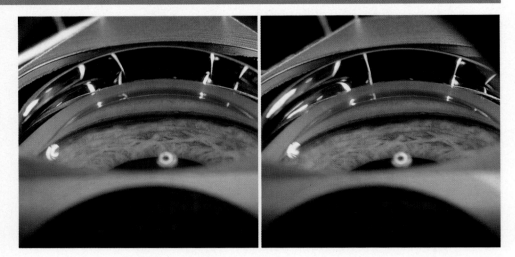

Figure shows the heavy degree of pigmentation that occurs within the trabecular meshwork in this syndrome. If one uses a grading scale from 0 to IV for the degree of pigmentation, with 0 being no pigmentation and the gradations in normal eyes running from 0 to II, pigmentary glaucoma usually falls into Grade III or more often Grade IV in regard to the degree of pigmentation. The pigment tends to collect over the posterior three-fifths of the trabecular meshwork, over Schlemm's canal, indicating that this is most likely the area of maximum flow through the trabecular meshwork to the canal. Occasionally, the anterior two-fifths of the meshwork will fill in as well. Pigment often collects along or anterior to Schwalbe's line, particularly inferiorly.

Fig. 5-7

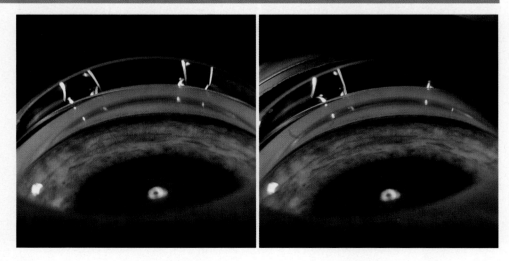

Figure shows the heavy degree of pigmentation that occurs within the trabecular meshwork in this syndrome. See Fig. 5-6 for description of grading scale.

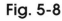

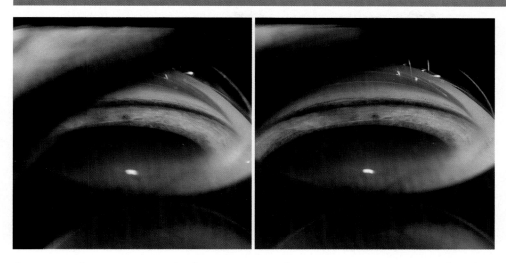

An unusual situation in which a patient with posterior iris concavity has lost the concavity in full dilation because the iris has lifted off the anterior lens surface. The lifting of the iris off the lens interrupts the inverse pupillary block and causes the iris to flatten.

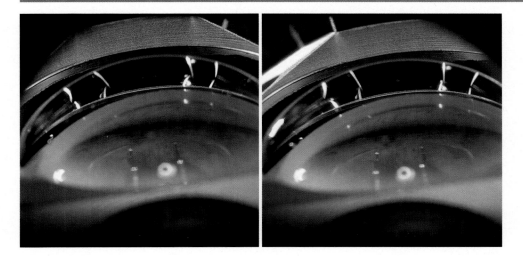

The anterior chamber, an angle of an eye in a patient who had an early, iris clip–type of intraocular lens. The lens caused chafing of the posterior surface of the iris that led to a secondary pigmentary glaucoma.

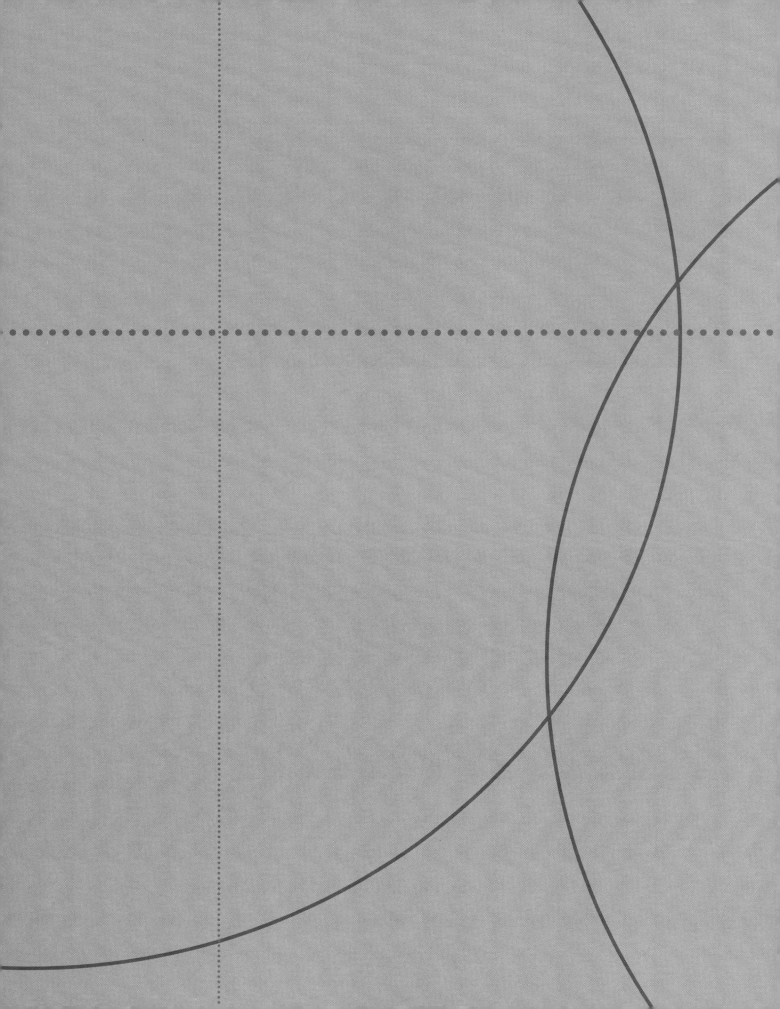

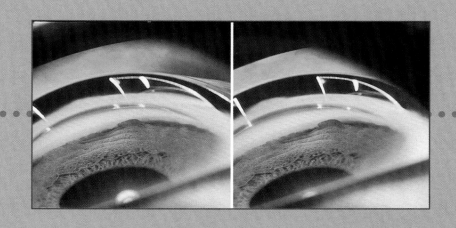

C H A P T E R   6

UVEITIC GLAUCOMA

Uveitis can cause glaucoma in a number of ways. Initially, the inflammatory cells can obstruct the intertrabecular spaces of the trabecular meshwork, elevating intraocular pressure. This situation can be reversed with steroid therapy. Later, chronic scarring within the trabecular meshwork can cause irreversible damage and elevation of intraocular pressure that will not respond favorably to steroid therapy. These are open-angle uveitic processes.

In some cases, inflammatory precipitates occur within the angle and on the trabecular meshwork. This inflammatory process may ultimately lead to irreversible synechial angle closure.

In other cases, the pupillary margin of the iris may completely seal to the anterior lens surface, preventing the forward passage of aqueous and causing iris bombé — a characteristic forward bulging of the iris that is highest at its central portion. The peripheral bulging can close the angle, causing first appositional closure and later synechial closure.

The intraocular pressure is always a measure of the balance between aqueous inflow and the resistance in the outflow channels. Uveoscleral outflow also may vary during an inflammatory episode. Aqueous production can remain normal during inflammation, or it can decrease, occasionally accounting for a lower than expected intraocular pressure that may rise if inflow normalizes.

SUGGESTED READINGS

Allingham RR: Glaucoma due to intraocular inflammation. In Epstein DL, Allingham RR, and Schuman JS, editors: Chandler and Grant's glaucoma, ed 4, Baltimore, 1997, Williams & Wilkins, pp 375–394.

Alward WLM: Color atlas of gonioscopy, London, England, 1994, Wolfe Publishing (Mosby-Year Book Europe Limited), pp 83, 86, 95–98.

Hoskins HD Jr and Kass MA: Secondary open-angle glaucoma. In Becker-Shaffer's diagnosis and therapy of the glaucomas, ed 6, St. Louis, 1989, Mosby-Year Book, Inc, pp 332–335.

Johnson D, Liesegang TJ, and Brubaker RF: Aqueous humor dynamics in Fuchs' uveitis syndrome. Am J Ophthalmol 95:783, 1983.

Krupin T, Feitl ME, and Karalekas D: Glaucoma associated with uveitis. In Ritch R, Shields MB, and Krupin T, editors: The glaucomas, ed 2, St. Louis, 1996, Mosby-Year Book, Inc, pp 1225–1258.

Mermoud A et al: [Prostaglandins E2 and F2-alpha in uveitic glaucoma in the Lewis rat]. Klin Monatsbl Augenheilkd 206:409, 1995.

Mermoud A et al: Animal model for uveitic glaucoma. Graefes Arch Clin Exp Ophthalmol 232:553, 1994.

Panek WC et al: Glaucoma in patients with uveitis. Br J Ophthalmol 74:223, 1990.

Roth M and Simmons RJ: Glaucoma associated with precipitates on the trabecular meshwork. Ophthalmology 86:1613, 1979.

Samples JR: Management of glaucoma secondary to uveitis. Am Acad Ophthalmol Focal Points XIII(5), June, 1995.

Fig. 6-1

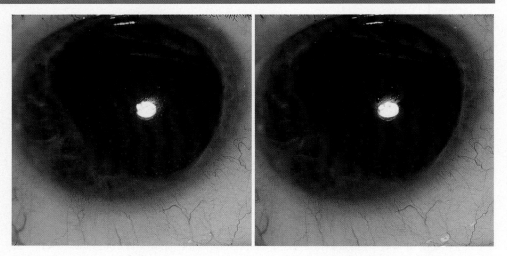

Keratic precipitates can be seen on the endothelium of this patient with granulomatous uveitis. If keratic precipitates are seen on the endothelium, particularly in the presence of elevated intraocular pressure, the trabecular meshwork should be inspected carefully for precipitates as well.

Fig. 6-2

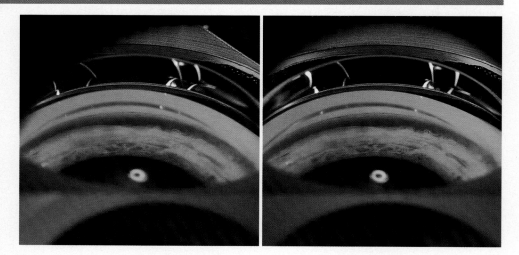

Keratic precipitates on the trabecular meshwork. Goniophotograph of a patient with confluent keratic precipitates covering the entire trabecular meshwork and ending at Schwalbe's line. Early congealing can be seen in the angle to the right. This patient was originally thought to have chronic open-angle glaucoma until accurate gonioscopy was performed.

Fig. 6-3

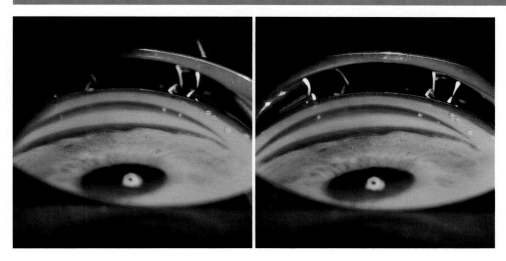

Goniophotograph of inflammatory infiltration of the trabecular meshwork that is not obvious except centrally, where a keratic precipitate dips down and is pathognomonic. Early synechia formation adjacent to the ciliary body band can be seen on each side of the keratic precipitate, and synechia formation to the trabecular meshwork can be seen on the far right.

Fig. 6-4

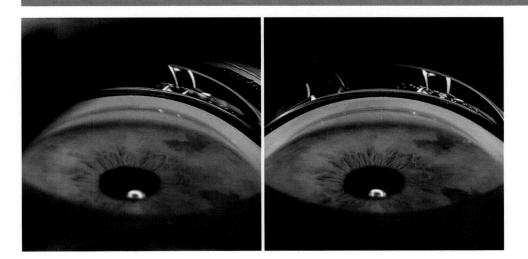

Goniophotograph of inflammation of the trabecular meshwork without specific or individual keratic precipitates seen. Here the trabecular meshwork lacks normal definition and detail, and early synechia formation can be seen to the right.

Fig. 6-5

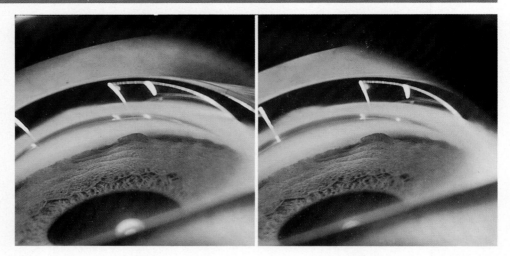

Goniophotograph of keratic precipitate of the trabecular meshwork hanging down centrally and to the right, with complete trabecular meshwork involvement and synechia formation to the mid–trabecular meshwork on the left and almost to Schwalbe's line on the right.

Fig. 6-6

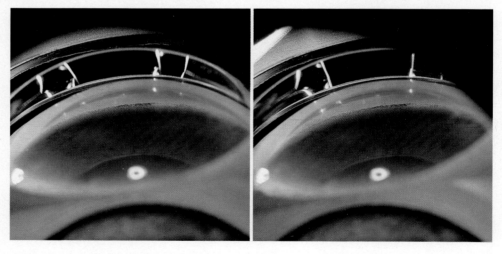

Goniophotograph of a patient with generalized inflammatory involvement of the trabecular meshwork to Schwalbe's line, without distinct keratic precipitates and with synechia formation only on the left.

Fig. 6-7

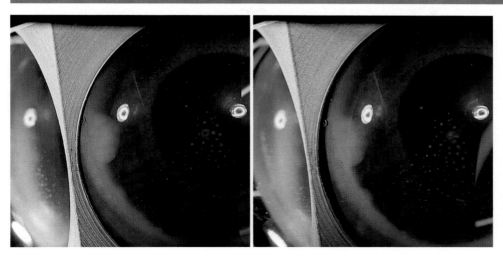

A combination anterior segment and goniophotograph of a patient with sarcoidosis with granulomatous endothelial keratic precipitates and multisized, whitish inflammatory nodules in the angle.

Fig. 6-8

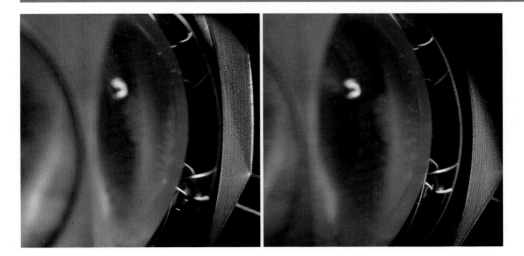

Goniophotograph of same patient as in Fig. 6-7, showing a large inflammatory nodule in the angle.

Fig. 6-9

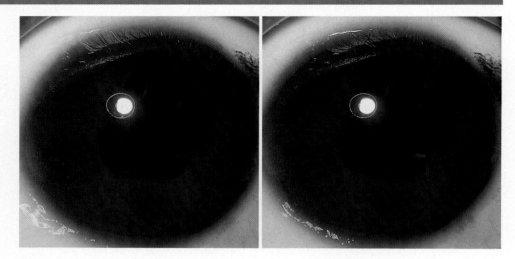

Anterior segment photograph of patient with inflammatory synechia formation to the lens inferiorly and to the left. Dilation of the pupil reveals an area without synechiae formation up and to the right, preventing a secluded pupil and iris bombé formation.

Fig. 6-10

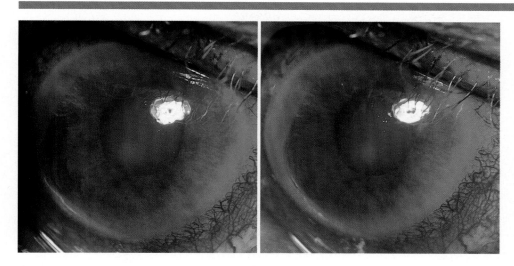

Anterior segment photograph illustrating iris bombé configuration of the iris with complete pupillary border synechia formation (secluded pupil) to a white and cataractous lens. Note the dome-like configuration to the iris with the highest point central.

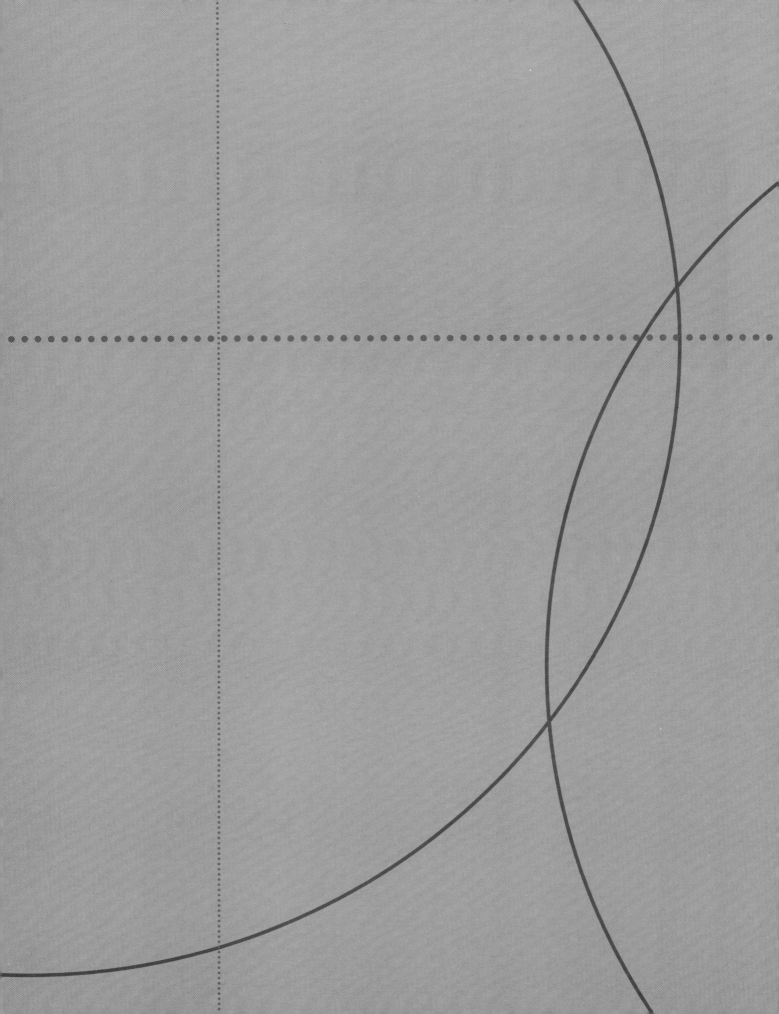

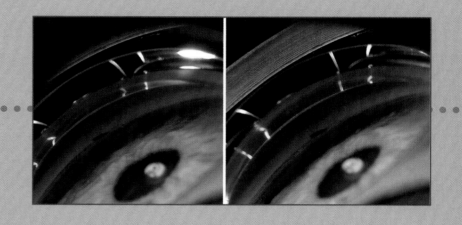

CHAPTER 7

TRAUMA

Blunt trauma to the anterior segment of the eye typically causes tearing of tissue within the anterior segment. Some of this tearing can be associated with development of various types of glaucoma.

There are seven rings of tissue that characteristically tear anterior to the equator after blunt anterior segment trauma. The seven rings should be examined in order. (1) The first ring that can tear is the pupillary margin, where small radial tears can be seen. The next six peripheral rings all tear in a concentric fashion. (2) The second ring of tissue that can tear is the base of the iris, resulting in a traumatic iridodialysis. The base of the iris at its insertion into the ciliary body is the thinnest portion of the iris. (3) The third ring that can tear is the ciliary body face itself, and in this circumferential tearing, the iris root is displaced posteriorly, resulting in angle recession. (4) The fourth ring of tissue that can tear is the trabecular meshwork. Here, circumferential tears within the tissue can be seen with careful examination. It is possible that tearing of the trabecular meshwork with subsequent scarring leads to the glaucoma formation associated with angle recession. (5) The fifth ring of tissue that can tear is at the insertion of the ciliary body into the scleral spur. When this tissue tears, a traumatic cyclodialysis cleft results. (6) The sixth ring of tissue that can tear is the zonular ring supporting the lens. Tearing of this tissue can result in lens subluxation or dislocation. (7) The seventh ring that can tear is the attachment of the retina at the ora seratta, resulting in retinal dialysis and detachment.

Traumatic bleeding into the anterior chamber typically results from tearing into the ciliary body face, which stretches and tears angle vessels.

Occasionally, trauma to the angle region can result in hemorrhage within the trabecular meshwork. Sometimes severe angle damage can result in a limited internal fibrous ingrowth from the torn angle into the anterior chamber.

The illustrations include a view of a partial hyphema, a total hyphema, views of tearing of the pupillary margin, a traumatic iridodialysis, various angle recessions, acute tearing into the trabecular meshwork itself, a traumatic cyclodialysis cleft, zonular ring rupture with lens subluxation, traumatic hemorrhage within the trabecular meshwork, limited internal fibrous ingrowth after severe angle damage, and a view of traumatic corneal blood staining. Pigment balls on the trabecular meshwork after the resolution of a hyphema often are seen. Such collections of pigment, often oval or round, are pathognomonic of the prior presence of a hyphema.

Ghost cell glaucoma can occur after trauma if there is a disruption in the anterior hyaloid face associated with vitreous hemorrhage. In the vitreous, a week or two after the injury, erythrocytes degenerate to ghost cells, which are khaki-colored (not red) and nonpliant. The ghost cells can pass forward into the anterior chamber through the anterior hyaloid face disruption, forming a khaki line in the anterior chamber. Sometimes severe obstruction to outflow results because the nonpliant ghost cells have difficulty passing through the trabecular meshwork.

In the traumatic carotid cavernous sinus fistula syndrome, arterialization of the venous drainage from the eye and from Schlemm's canal can result in dilation of conjunctival and episcleral veins and elevation of pressure within Schlemm's canal. Occasionally, blood reflux causes increased resistance to outflow and elevation of the intraocular pressure.

SUGGESTED READINGS

Campbell DG: Ghost cell glaucoma following trauma, Ophthalmology 88:1151, 1981.

Campbell DG: Iris retraction associated with rhegmatogenous retinal detachment syndrome and hypotony: a new explanation. Arch Ophthalmol 102:1457, 1984.

Campbell DG: Traumatic glaucoma. In Shingleton BJ, Hersh PS, and Kenyon KR, editors: Eye trauma, St. Louis, 1991, Mosby-Year Book, Inc, pp 117–125.

Campbell DG and Essigmann EM: Hemolytic ghost cell glaucoma: further studies. Arch Ophthalmol 97:2141, 1979.

Campbell DG and Schertzer RM: Ghost cell glaucoma. In Ritch R, Shields MB, and Krupin T, editors: The glaucomas, ed 2, St. Louis, 1996, Mosby-Year Book, Inc, pp 1277–1285.

Epstein DL: Cyclodialysis. In Epstein DL, Allingham RR, and Schuman JS, editors: Chandler and Grant's glaucoma, ed 4, Baltimore, 1997, Williams & Wilkins, pp 573–579.

Hoskins HD Jr and Kass MA: Secondary open-angle glaucoma. In Becker-Shaffer's diagnosis and therapy of the glaucomas, ed 6, St. Louis, 1989, Mosby-Year Book, Inc, pp 324–330.

Mermoud A and Heuer DK: Glaucoma associated with trauma. In Ritch R, Shields MB, and Krupin T, editors: The glaucomas, ed 2, St. Louis, 1996, Mosby-Year Book, Inc, pp 1259–1275.

Shingleton BJ: Glaucoma due to trauma. In Epstein DL, Allingham RR, and Schuman JS, editors: Chandler and Grant's glaucoma, ed 4, Baltimore, 1997, Williams & Wilkins, pp 395–403.

Tingey DP and Shingleton BJ: Glaucoma associated with ocular trauma. In Albert DM and Jakobiec FA, editors: Principles and practice of ophthalmology, Philadelphia, 1993, WB Saunders Co, pp 1436–1444.

Fig. 7-1

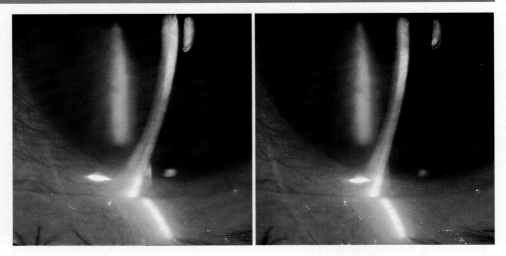

A slit-lamp photograph of a small, fresh hyphema that has layered inferiorly.

Fig. 7-2

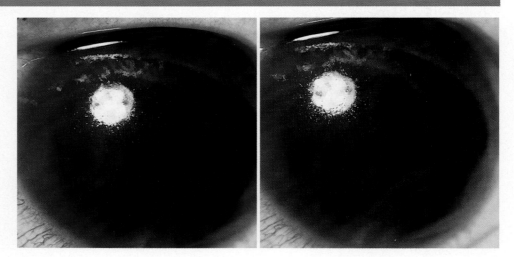

A complete, or eight-ball, hyphema that demonstrates the darkened and purplish color of a complete hyphema. With a complete hyphema, the intraocular pressure often can elevate to very high levels. Corneal blood staining (see Fig. 7-17) must be diligently searched for.

Fig. 7-3

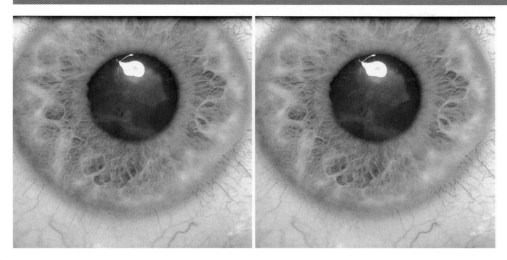

A patient who has had blunt anterior segment trauma. A small radial tear into the pupillary margin is visible at 9 o'clock. This represents the first ring that can tear. Corneal and anterior lenticular scarring also are visible.

Fig. 7-4

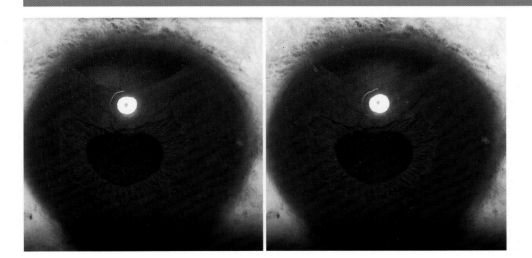

A superior, traumatic iridodialysis with characteristic deformation of the pupil, the second ring that can tear.

Fig. 7-5

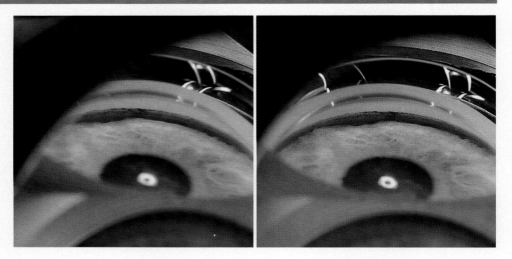

A mild angle recession with irregularity of the width of the ciliary body band, with slight traumatic synechia formation just left of the widest portion of the band (same eye as in Fig. 7.3). Tearing of the ciliary body face represents the third ring that can tear.

Fig. 7-6

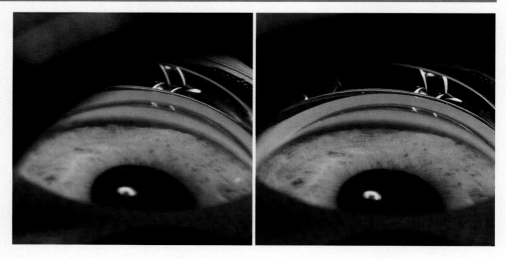

A mild angle recession inferiorly and to the left, compared with a more normal-appearing angle inferiorly and to the right. There is a small collection of pigment on the ciliary body band that appears oval. Pigment balls are pathognomonic of a previous hyphema.

Fig. 7-7

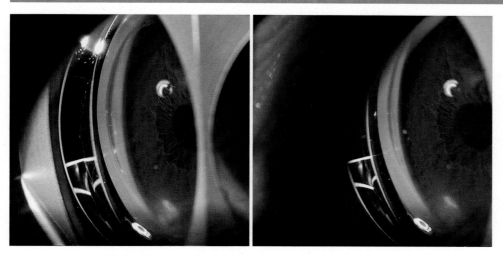

A gonioscopic view of the same eye depicted in Fig. 7-4, showing the gradual development of angle recession. Angle recession starts from the bottom, where the angle is almost normal, up to the top where the ciliary body band is widened considerably. The iris is then completely torn away as the iridodialysis begins.

Fig. 7-8

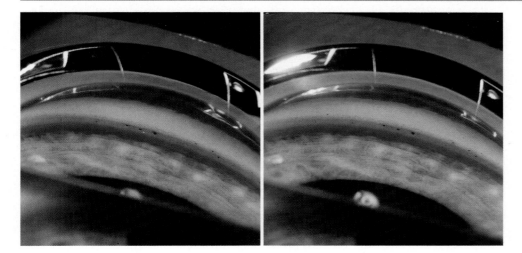

A gonioscopic view of a marked traumatic angle recession, showing the ciliary body band to be wider than the trabecular meshwork itself — an abnormal finding. Small pigment balls are visible on the trabecular meshwork, and circumferential tears can be seen in the face of the ciliary body below and just to the right of the large, central pigment ball, and again further to the right. These pigment balls indicate a previous hyphema.

Fig. 7-9

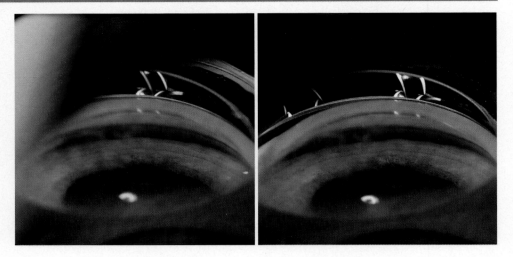

Extensive angle recession with marked widening of the ciliary body band throughout. There is pigmentation of the trabecular meshwork and a slightly whitish line suggesting the scleral spur below it, and then a large area of bare ciliary body. On the pupillary margin, there is a small area of iris atrophy as well.

Fig. 7-10

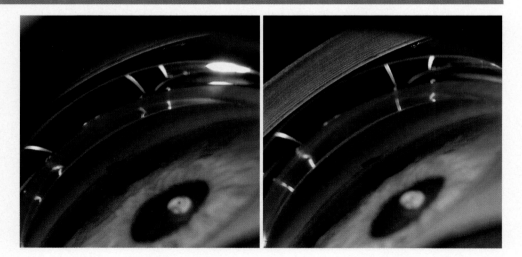

A goniophotograph of extensive and obvious angle recession everywhere, with a smooth, bare ciliary body band on the left and on the right, adjacent to the iris root. Note the large tear in the trabecular meshwork itself: Torn tissue has folded over the scleral spur region in the straight-ahead position. A large patch of flattened pigment covers the tear and appears to hold the torn tissue in place. The meshwork is torn to the left of this pigment as well. There are other flattened collections of pigment, along with balls of pigment, all pathognomonic of a prior hyphema.

Fig. 7-11

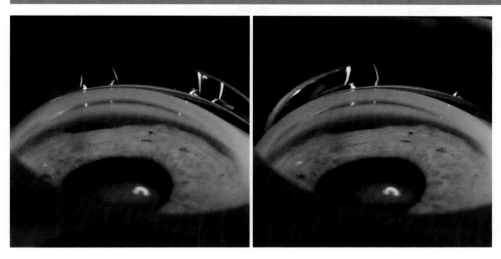

A goniophotograph showing an area of angle recession in the straight-ahead position. A small area of iridodialysis exposing individual ciliary processes also is visible. This demonstrates that an iridodialysis can extend from an area of an angle recession.

Fig. 7-12

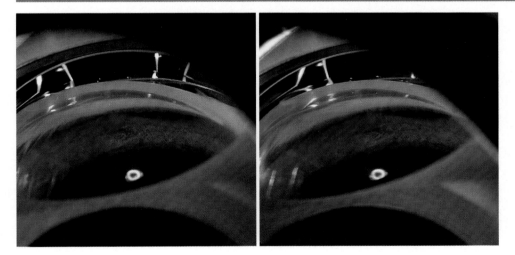

A goniophotograph of the fourth ring of tissue that can tear. This shows a cyclodialysis cleft, toward the right, indicating that the ciliary body has torn off the scleral spur. Fluid now has access to the suprachoroidal space from the anterior chamber. This often results in profound hypotony. An area of synechial scarring to the trabecular meshwork can be seen to the left of the cleft. Gray iris atrophy occurs below the cleft.

Fig. 7-13

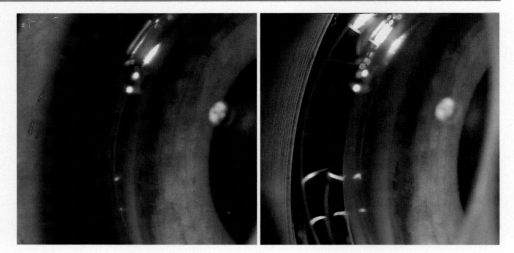

Goniophotograph indicating the fifth ring of tissue that can tear, the trabecular meshwork. This photograph, taken soon after the injury, shows partial resolution of hemorrhage. A tear in the trabecular meshwork itself is visible, with torn tissue rolled in the scleral spur region centrally. There is associated angle recession below the torn trabecular meshwork as well.

Fig. 7-14

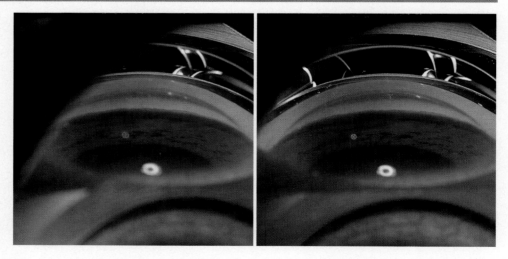

Goniophotograph of a rare finding — traumatic hemorrhage within the trabecular meshwork itself.

Fig. 7-15

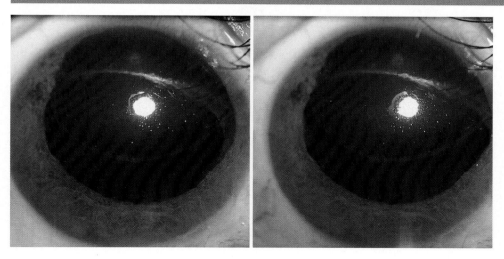

An anterior segment photograph of a patient after blunt injury to the eye, showing tearing of the sixth ring of tissue, the zonular ring, with superior dislocation of the lens. In this situation, vitreous has herniated forward inferiorly, and angle closure also has developed.

Fig. 7-16

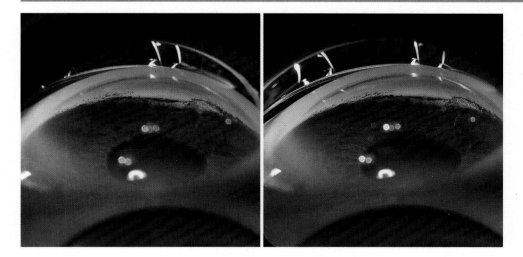

A goniophotograph showing a rare complication of traumatic damage to the angle with limited fibrous ingrowth into the angle.

Fig. 7-17

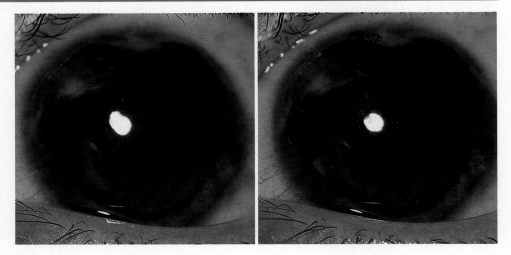

Corneal blood staining after complete hyphema.

Fig. 7-18

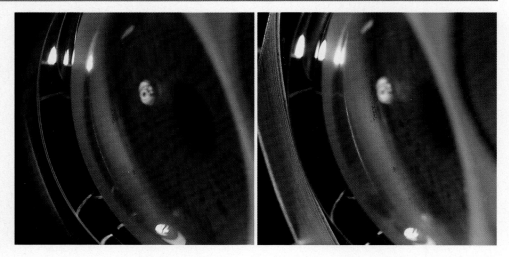

A goniophotograph showing the appearance of a trabecular meshwork after direct blunt traumatic damage. The torn edges have smoothed out, leaving a mild depression or indentation in the trabecular meshwork in the region where there is deposition of pigment as well.

Fig. 7-19

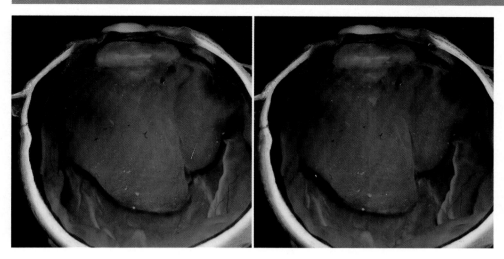

Pathologic specimen of a patient with ghost cell glaucoma that originated from a vitreous hemorrhage. The characteristic khaki color of the degenerated erythrocytes and their products can be seen. The posterior hyaloid face has detached.

Fig. 7-20

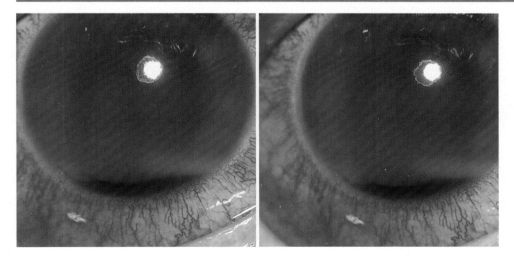

An anterior segment photograph of a patient with ghost cell glaucoma approximately 2 weeks after blunt traumatic hyphema formation with vitreous hemorrhage. The hyphema, the purple layer at bottom, has almost resolved, but now the anterior chamber contains a profusion of ghost cells that have passed forward from the vitreous. A layer of khaki cells is beginning to form on the hyphema layer. The khaki color is pathgonomonic and can be distinguished easily from a white layer of leukocytes (hypopyon).

Fig. 7-21

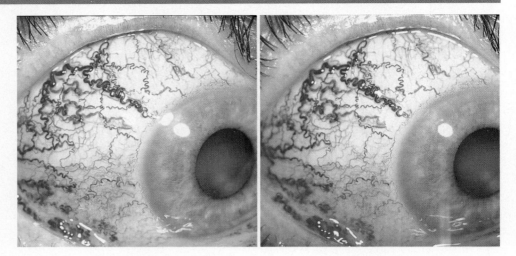

An anterior segment photograph in a patient with traumatic carotid cavernous sinus fistula showing extreme and tortuous dilation of conjunctival and episcleral vessels.

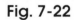

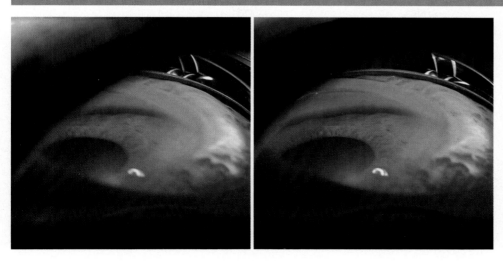

A goniophotograph of a different patient with a traumatic carotid cavernous sinus fistula. Dilated surface veins are apparent, along with a faint, reddish blush in the trabecular meshwork to the right indicating secondary blood reflux into Schlemm's canal.

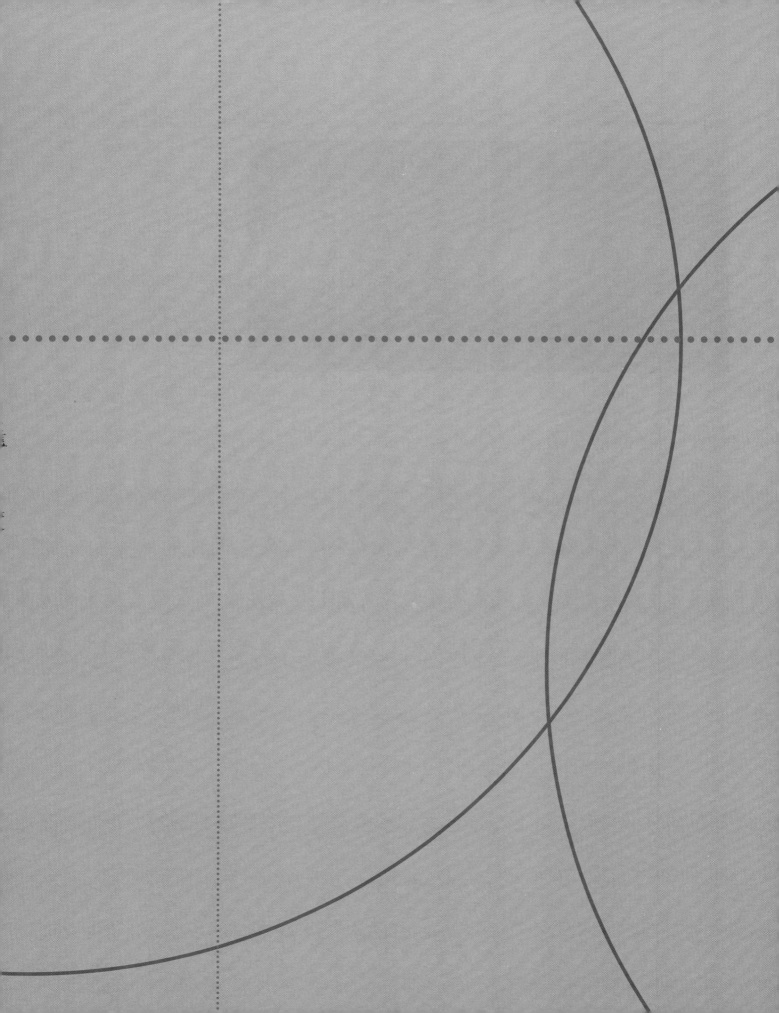

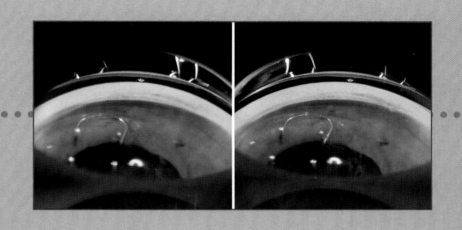

CHAPTER 8

LENS-INDUCED GLAUCOMA

In phacolytic glaucoma, a cataractous, hypermature lens develops with cortical liquefaction. The liquefied material can leak through the capsule, causing a vigorous macrophage response in the anterior chamber. The trabecular meshwork can become severely obstructed by material leaking from the lens.

Patients with phacomorphic glaucoma present with an intumescent cataract, shallowing of the anterior chamber, a closed angle, and elevated intraocular pressure. Rarely, a lens can dislocate into the anterior chamber, causing a pupillary block anterior to the pupillary margin, and a secondary angle-closure glaucoma.

Anterior chamber intraocular lenses occasionally can cause irritation within the anterior segment, resulting in uveitis-glaucoma-hyphema syndrome.

Posterior iris chafing by an improperly positioned posterior chamber intraocular lens can cause a secondary pigmentary glaucoma. Iris clip lenses, implanted during a previous era of intraocular lens development, also can cause secondary pigmentary glaucoma.

SUGGESTED READINGS

Brooks AM, Grant G, and Gillies WE: Comparison of specular microscopy and examination of aspirate in phacolytic glaucoma. Ophthalmology 97:85, 1990.

Campbell DG and Schertzer RM: Pigmentary glaucoma. In Ritch R, Shields MB, and Krupin T, editors: The glaucomas, ed 2, St. Louis, 1996, Mosby-Year Book, Inc, pp 975–991.

Epstein DL: Lens-induced glaucoma. In Epstein DL, Allingham RR, and Schuman JS, editors: Chandler and Grant's glaucoma, ed 4, Baltimore, 1997, Williams & Wilkins, pp 422–430.

Epstein DL, Jedziniak JA, and Grant WM: Obstruction of aqueous outflow by lens particles and by heavy-molecular-weight soluble lens proteins. Invest Ophthalmol Vis Sci 17: 272, 1978.

Flocks M, Littwin CS, and Zimmerman LE: Phacolytic glaucoma: clinicopathologic study of 138 cases of glaucoma associated with hypermature cataract. Arch Ophthalmol 54:37, 1955.

Hoskins HB Jr and Kass MA: Secondary open-angle glaucoma. In Becker-Shaffer's diagnosis and therapy of the glaucomas, ed 6, St. Louis, 1989, Mosby-Year Book, Inc, pp 316–324.

Liebmann JM and Ritch R: Glaucoma associated with lens intumescence and dislocation. In Ritch R, Shields MB, and Krupin T, editors: The glaucomas, ed 2, St. Louis, 1996, Mosby-Year Book, Inc, pp 1033–1053.

Richter CU: Lens-induced open-angle glaucoma. In Ritch R, Shields MB, and Krupin T, editors: The glaucomas, ed 2, St. Louis, 1996, Mosby-Year Book, Inc, pp 1023–1031.

Tomey KF and Traverso CE: Glaucoma associated with aphakia and pseudophakia. In Ritch R, Shields MB, and Krupin T, editors: The glaucomas, ed 2, St. Louis, 1996, Mosby-Year Book, Inc, pp 1289–1323.

Ueno H et al: Electron microscopic observation of the cells floating in the anterior chamber in a case of phacolytic glaucoma. Jpn J Ophthalmol 33:103, 1989.

Fig. 8-1

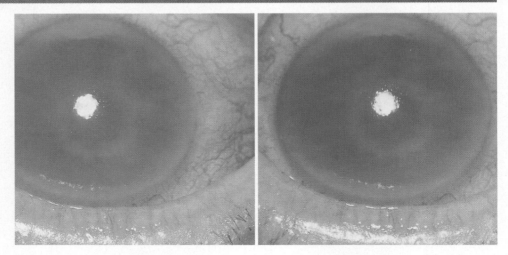

A patient with phacolytic glaucoma, a sudden elevation of intraocular pressure in association with hypermature lens obscured by severe secondary corneal edema.

Fig. 8-2

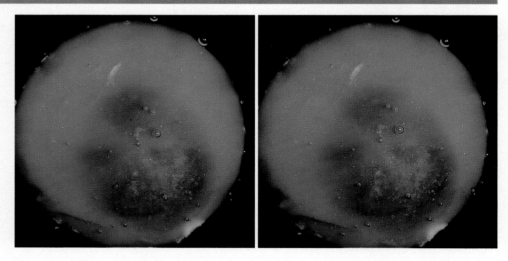

A hypermature lens removed via intracapsular cataract extraction showing a mobile, dark brown nucleus floating in white, liquefied cortical material.

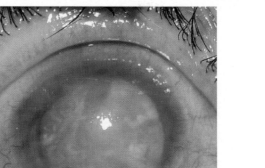

Fig. 8-3

Anterior segment photograph showing a mature lens that has dislocated into the anterior chamber, causing a pupillary block with peripheral iris bulging and angle closure.

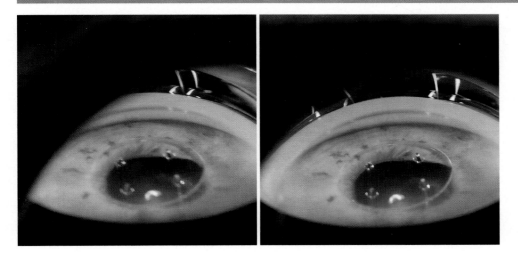

Fig. 8-4

The uveitis-glaucoma-hyphema syndrome. A goniophotograph of an early model, iris clip–type intraocular lens with inflammatory obscuration of the trabecular meshwork.

Fig. 8-5

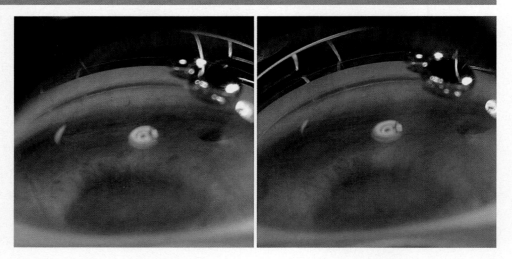

The uveitis-glaucoma-hyphema syndrome. A goniophotograph of an anterior chamber intraocular lens with keratic precipitates on the lens. Two footplates can be seen indenting the ciliary body band.

Fig. 8-6

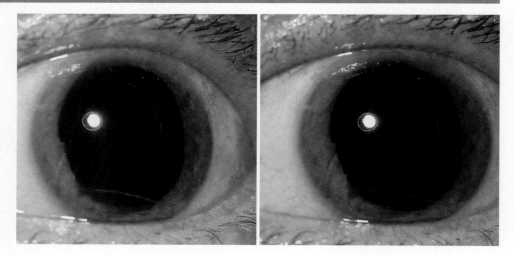

The uveitis-glaucoma-hyphema syndrome. An anterior segment view of an anterior chamber intraocular lens associated with a small hyphema.

Fig. 8-7

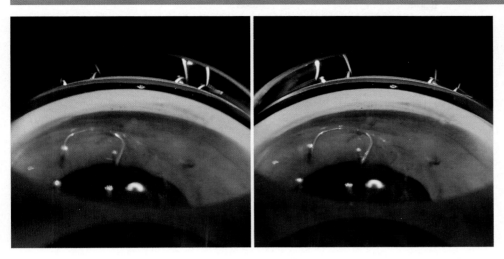

Goniophotograph of a patient with secondary pigmentary glaucoma due to posterior iris chafing, in this case by an iris clip–type intraocular lens that has dislocated into the anterior chamber inferiorly. The dark pigment band within the trabecular meshwork is visible just inferiorly.

Fig. 8-8

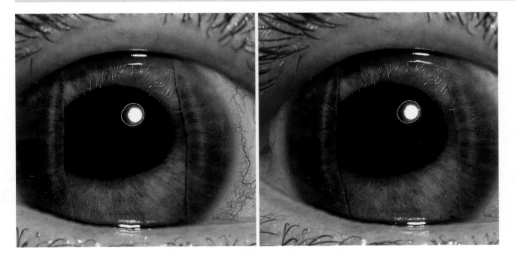

Anterior segment photograph of a plate anterior chamber intraocular lens with pupillary block and severe peripheral iris bulging with angle closure.

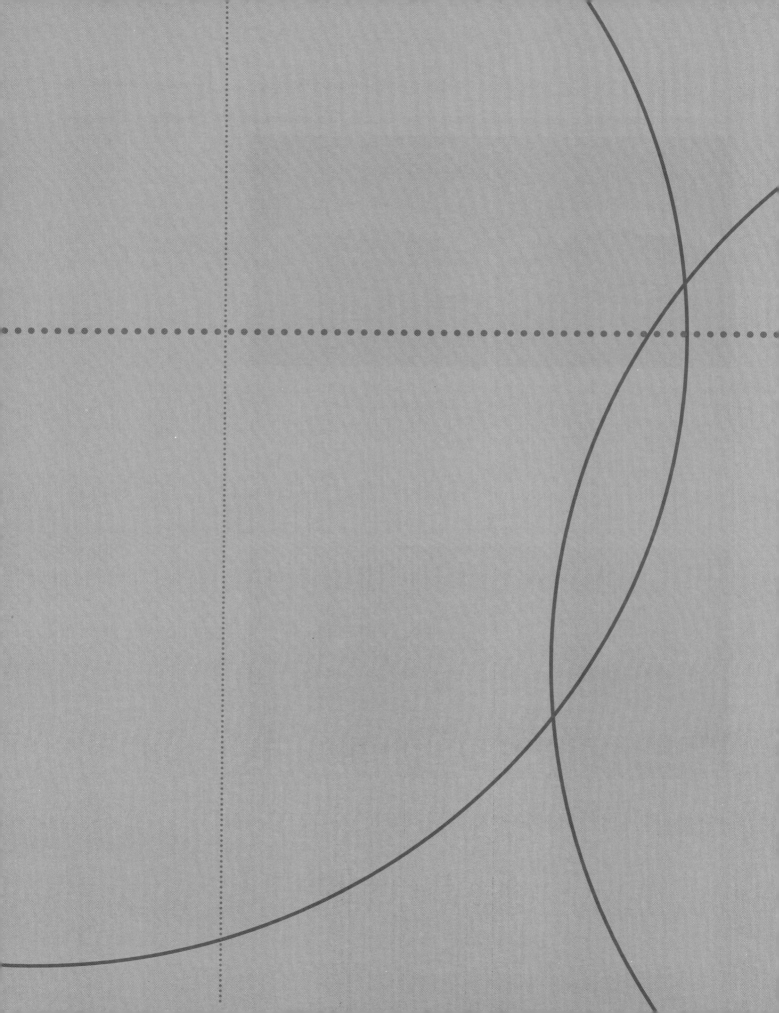

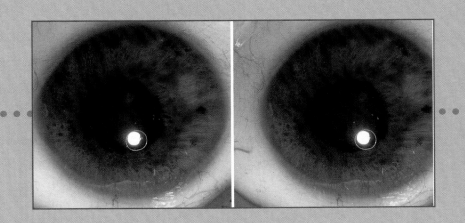

CHAPTER 9

THE IRIDO-CORNEAL-
ENDOTHELIAL SYNDROME

The ocular disease first called essential iris atrophy and two closely associated syndromes, the Cogan–Reese syndrome and Chandler syndrome, have been referred to more recently in a group as the irido-corneal-endothelial (ICE) syndrome.

This spectrum of diseases can best be understood if one understands that ICE syndrome begins as a rare, unilateral, degenerative disease of the corneal endothelium. In the classic form of the disease, the changes in the cornea are initially and primarily proliferative. The corneal endothelium abnormally proliferates over the trabecular meshwork and out onto the surface of the iris. The development of an abnormal Descemet's membrane is associated with the proliferation of the endothelial cells. The abnormal proliferation is contractile, and contraction within the angle region can lead to small, tent-like areas of angle closure that can grow until the entire angle becomes closed permanently and synechially. Occasionally, the membrane will overgrow the open angle without synechia formation. As the membrane extends onto the surface of the iris, it continues to contract, sometimes causing severe corectopia. Contraction of the membrane also may cause ectropion uveae. Occasionally, as the membrane grows across the surface of the iris, it leaves islands of normal iris tissue behind that are then enveloped as the membrane squeezes these islands, pushing them up into small nodules. Eventually, the membrane entirely covers the nodules.

The membrane can grow in one portion of the angle, or it can grow in different portions. If a membrane has grown in one portion of the angle and has pulled the iris toward that area, and if another membrane grows in the approximately opposite angle, the contraction will exceed the ability of the iris to stretch. Large separation or stretch holes will form in the iris as the iris literally tears through both the stroma and the pigment epithelium. Occasionally, the contraction within the region of peripheral anterior synechia formation will constrict and occlude the radial iris vessels that feed the iris internally, and small, oval, ischemic atrophy holes will develop. These holes appear different from the often larger stretch holes that can occur.

The elevation of intraocular pressure that can be associated with this disease is caused by the coverage of the trabecular meshwork by the membrane and by the secondary synechia formation. Later in the disease process, the endothelium can degenerate as well, allowing corneal edema to develop, often at pressures that would not ordinarily cause corneal edema.

In Chandler syndrome, which is a variant of this disease process, the degeneration of the corneal endothelium is much greater. The degenerating cells allow corneal edema at pressures that would not ordinarily cause edema, sometimes even at normal intraocular pressure. The cells tend not to proliferate as vigorously as in essential iris atrophy, but there usually is local proliferation over the angle with contraction and corectopia and occasionally some of the other signs of the disease. At this end of the spectrum of the disease, however, one can characterize the process as being more degenerative and less proliferative, whereas at the essential iris atrophy end of the spectrum, one can characterize the process as being less degenerative and more proliferative.

The Cogan–Reese syndrome, which is associated with peripheral anterior synechia formation and extensive iris nodule formation, is included in this spectrum of diseases when nodule formation occurs. Nodules develop in only a small percentage of patients with essential iris atrophy.

The peripheral anterior synechiae that develop in this syndrome are pathognomonic because they are yellowish and extend onto the surface of the corneal endothelium beyond Schwalbe's line, an extension that is unusual for many other synechial syndromes.

Recent studies have indicated that this disease process may be viral. The disease process, now understood pathophysiologically, can best be characterized as a proliferative endotheliopathy. If a viral etiology is established absolutely, perhaps the entire disease process should be renamed viral proliferative endotheliopathy.

SUGGESTED READINGS

Alvarado JA et al: Detection of herpes simplex viral DNA in the iridocorneal endothelial syndrome. Arch Ophthalmol 112:1601, 1994.

Alward WLM: Color atlas of gonioscopy, London, England, 1994, Wolfe Publishing (Mosby-Year Book Europe Limited), pp 79–80.

Campbell DG, Shields MB, and Smith TR: The corneal endothelium and the spectrum of essential iris atrophy. Am J Ophthalmol 86:317, 1978.

Chandler PA: Atrophy of the stroma of the iris: endothelial dystrophy, corneal edema, and glaucoma. Am J Ophthalmol 41:607, 1956.

Cogan DG and Reese AB: A syndrome of iris nodules, ectopic Descemet's membrane, and unilateral glaucoma. Doc Ophthalmol 26:424, 1969.

Eagle RC Jr et al: Proliferative endotheliopathy with iris abnormalities: the iridocorneal endothelial syndrome. Arch Ophthalmol 97:2104, 1979.

Hoskins HD Jr and Kass MA: Angle closure glaucoma without pupillary block. In Becker-Shaffer's diagnosis and therapy of the glaucomas, ed 6, St. Louis, 1989, Mosby-Year Book, Inc, pp 248–252.

Huna R, Barak A, and Melamed S: Bilateral iridocorneal endothelial syndrome presented as Cogan-Reese and Chandler's syndrome. J Glaucoma 5:60, 1996.

Kupfer C et al: The contralateral eye in the iridocorneal endothelial (ICE) syndrome. Ophthalmology 90:1343, 1983.

Levy SG et al: Pathology of the iridocorneal-endothelial syndrome: the ICE-cell. Invest Ophthalmol Vis Sci 36:2592, 1995.

Shields MB: Iridocorneal endothelial syndromes. In Epstein DL, Allingham RR, and Schuman JS, editors: Chandler and Grant's glaucoma, ed 4, Baltimore, 1997, Williams & Wilkins, pp 319–326.

Shields MB and Bourgeois JE: Glaucoma associated with primary disorders of the corneal endothelium. In Ritch R, Shields MB, and Krupin T, editors: The glaucomas, ed 2, St. Louis, 1996, Mosby-Year Book, Inc, pp 957–974.

Shields MB, Campbell DG, and Simmons RJ: The essential iris atrophies. Am J Ophthalmol 85:749-1978.

Tsai CS et al: Antibodies to Epstein-Barr virus in iridocorneal endothelial syndrome. Arch Ophthalmol 108:1572, 1990.

Fig. 9-1

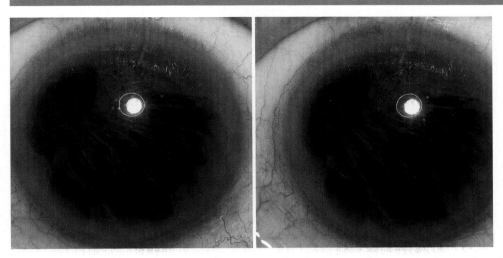

Anterior segment photograph of a patient with essential iris atrophy with a clear cornea, corectopia toward 10 o'clock, ectropion uveae in that direction, and central stretch holes centrally, indicating that peripheral anterior synechias exist at both the 4 o'clock and 10 o'clock regions. Fine iris nodules cover much of the iris surface, suggesting that an endothelial membrane has grown in these areas. The posterior pigment layer of the iris is exposed at the edge of the stretch holes, indicating that the iris has disintegrated from anterior to posterior.

Fig. 9-2

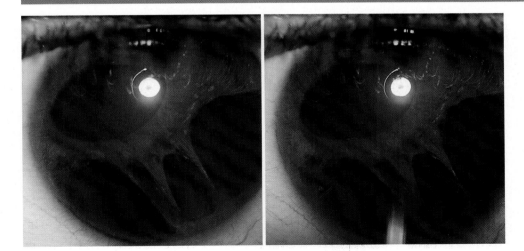

Anterior segment photograph of a different patient with essential iris atrophy, illustrating many of the same findings as in Fig. 9-1. No iris nodules are visible.

Fig. 9-3

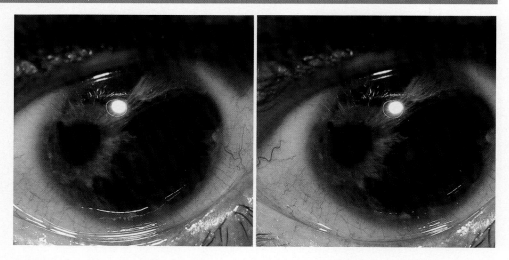

Anterior segment photograph of another patient with essential iris atrophy with corectopia toward 9 o'clock, illustrating high, yellowish, peripheral anterior synechiae, especially at the 8:30 and 9:30 positions. These synechiae are pathognomonic of the ICE syndrome.

Fig. 9-4

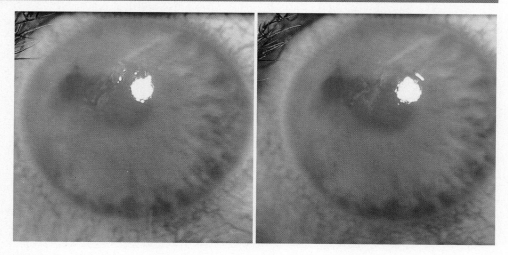

Chandler syndrome. An anterior segment photograph of a patient with severe corneal edema at a relatively low intraocular pressure with only mild signs of aberrant endothelial proliferation. Mild corectopia and ectropion uveae are visible toward 10 o'clock, with no iris hole formation.

Fig. 9-5

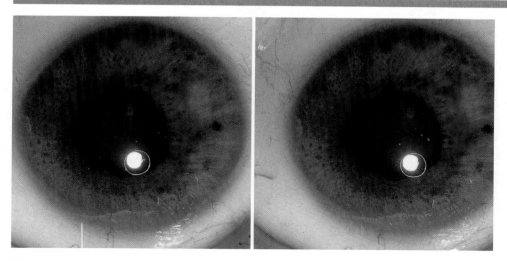

The iris nodule, or Cogan–Reese, syndrome. An anterior segment photograph of a patient with a high, yellowish, peripheral anterior synechia at 9 o'clock, pathognomonic of this syndrome. Round iris nodules to the right side of the iris indicate the presence of an endothelial membrane in this region.

Fig. 9-6

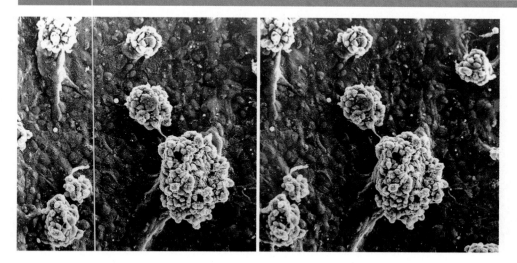

Stereo scanning electron micrograph of the same iris surface seen in Fig. 9-5. The iris surface is covered by an endothelial membrane that is growing up in stalklike fashion around islands of formerly normal iris tissue.

Fig. 9-7

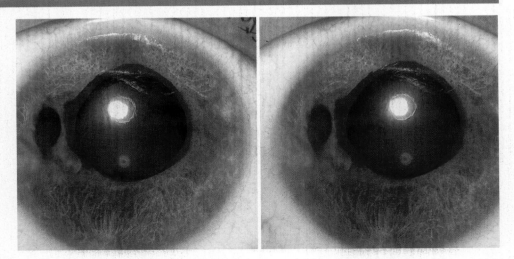

Anterior segment photograph of a patient with essential iris atrophy with peripheral anterior synechia formation in all quadrants, causing dilation of the pupil but leaving it relatively central. Severe synechia formation has caused an iris hole that is not the more common stretch hole but is rather the rarer atrophy hole.

Fig. 9-8

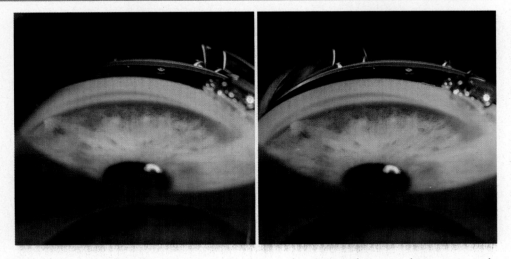

Goniophotograph of a patient with essential iris atrophy revealing very early tent-like peripheral anterior synechia formation — a process that can progress to close large portions of the angle.

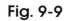

Fig. 9-9

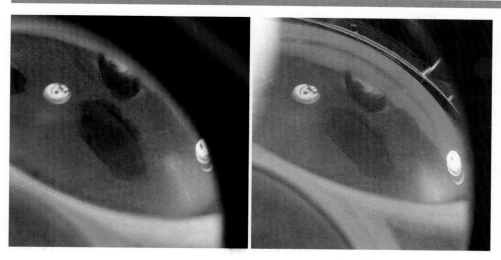

Goniophotograph of a patient with essential iris atrophy with complete, synechial angle-closure glaucoma with multiple iris nodules. Filtration surgery has been performed, and the internal opening of the sclerostomy can be seen above the surgically created peripheral iridectomy.

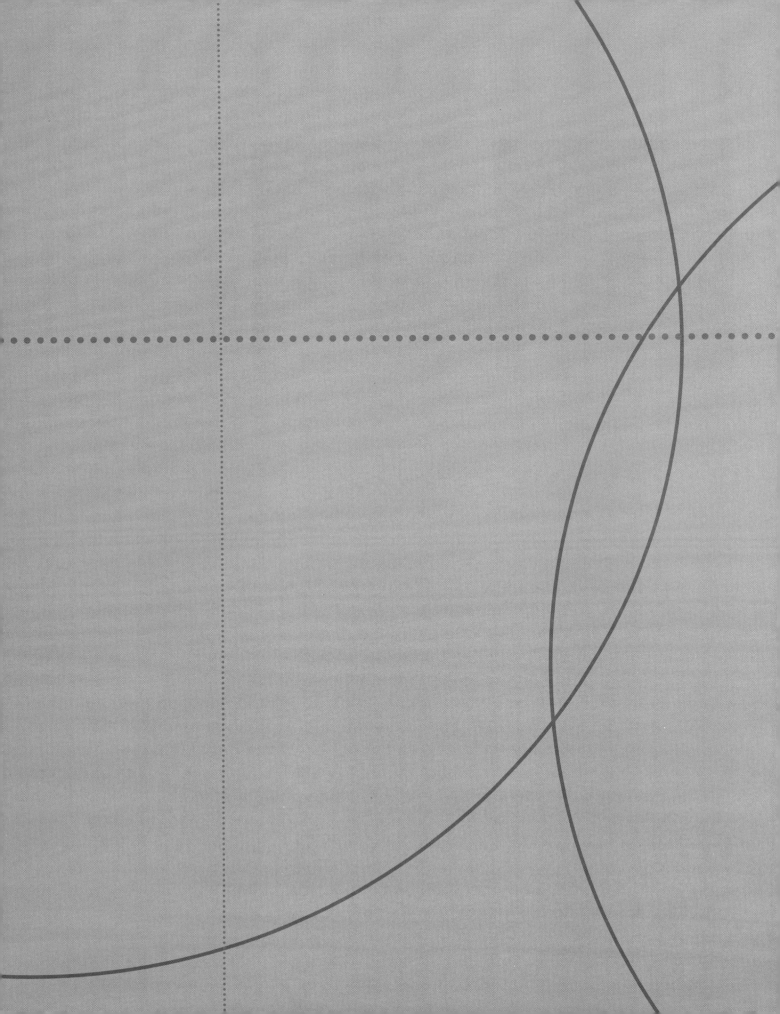

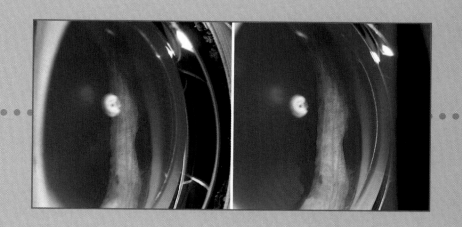

CHAPTER 10

TUMORS AND CYSTS

Intraocular tumors, primarily malignant melanomas, can present in the anterior chamber, in the posterior chamber, in the posterior segment of the eye, and occasionally in the angle first.

The tumors can fill the angle and cover the trabecular meshwork directly, causing glaucoma, or they can cause angle closure by pressing the lens forward if the tumor is posterior. Tumors also can shed cells and debris, which may obstruct the trabecular meshwork. Neovascular glaucoma also may be caused by intraocular tumors.

SUGGESTED READINGS

Alward WLM: Color atlas of gonioscopy, London, England, 1994, Wolfe Publishing (Mosby-Year Book Europe Limited), pp 105–106.

Duker JS: Glaucoma secondary to intraocular tumors. In Epstein DL, Allingham RR, and Schuman JS, editors: Chandler and Grant's glaucoma, ed 4, Baltimore, 1997, Williams & Wilkins, pp 366–371.

Hoskins HD Jr and Kass MA: Secondary open-angle glaucoma. In Becker-Shaffer's diagnosis and therapy of the glaucomas, ed 6, St. Louis, 1989, Mosby-Year Book, Inc, pp 335–336.

Narieman AN et al: Diffuse iris nevus manifested by unilateral open angle glaucoma. Ophthalmology 99:125, 1981.

Ozment R: Ocular tumors and glaucoma. In Albert DM and Jakobiec FA, editors: Principles and practice of ophthalmology, Philadelphia, 1994, WB Saunders Co, pp 1455–1462.

Shields CL et al: Prevalence and mechanism of secondary intraocular pressure elevation in eyes with intraocular tumors. Ophthalmology 94:839, 1987.

Shields JA, Annesley WH, and Spaeth GL: Necrotic melanocytoma of iris with secondary glaucoma. Am J Ophthalmol 84:826, 1977.

Shields JA and Shields CA: Intraocular tumors: a text and atlas, Philadelphia, 1992, WB Saunders Co, pp 11–43.

Shields JA et al: Metastatic tumors in the iris in 40 patients. Am J Ophthalmol 119:422, 1995.

Shields JA, Shields CL, and Shields MB: Glaucoma associated with intraocular tumors. In Ritch R, Shields MB, and Krupin T, editors: The glaucomas, ed 2, St. Louis, 1996, Mosby-Year Book, Inc, pp 1131–1139.

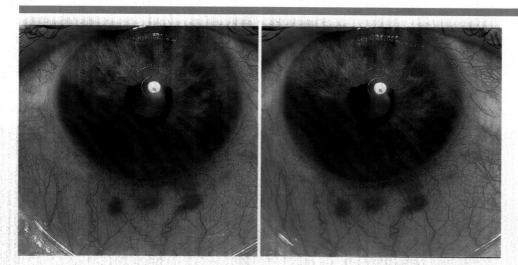

Fig. 10-1

Diffuse melanoma of the anterior iris surface. Anterior segment photograph of a diffuse iris melanoma involving most of the iris, sparing a small portion around 2 o'clock and causing ectropion uveae. In the angle a more solid mass can be seen, inferiorly, on the sclera. The brown dots indicate tumor growth out the collector channels from Schlemm's canal to the scleral surface.

Fig. 10-2

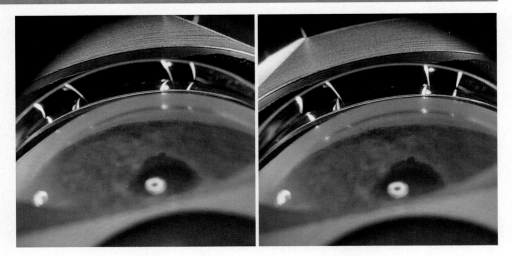

Goniophotograph of same patient as in Fig. 10-1 2 years later, showing diffuse angle involvement by tumor growth. This involvement causes severe elevation of intraocular pressure.

Fig. 10-3

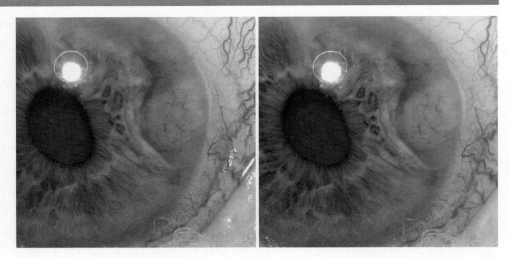

Anterior segment photograph of a patient with an amelanotic melanoma arising from the ciliary body and extending into the anterior chamber from the angle region. The adjacent surface vessels are dilated.

Fig. 10-4

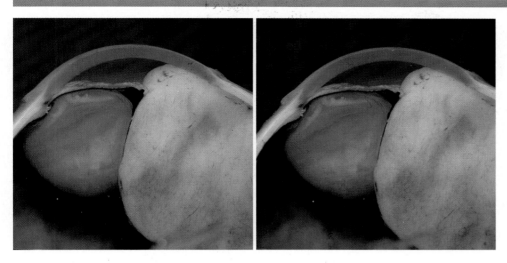

Gross pathologic cross section of the eye shown in Fig. 10-3 after enucle-
ation. The trabecular meshwork has been covered directly by the white tumor
on one side, and a secondary angle closure has occurred on the other side
due to lens deformation and displacement.

Fig. 10-5

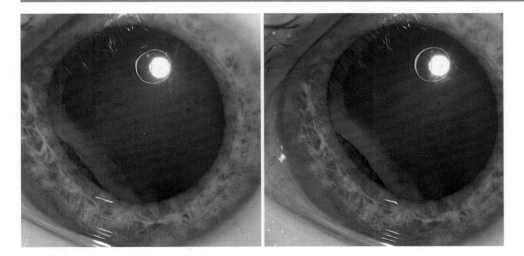

Anterior segment photograph of a malignant melanoma of the ciliary body
with tumor extension anteriorly into the angle at 7 o'clock.

Fig. 10-6

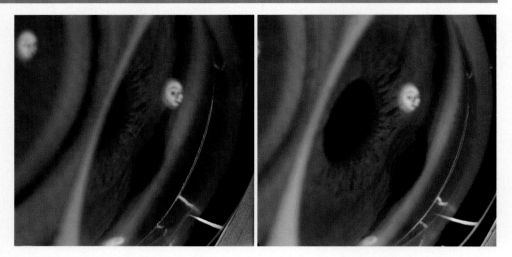

Goniophotograph of the angle of a patient with a malignant melanoma of the ciliary body that has extended anteriorly into the angle. Superior to the tumor, Schlemm's canal has filled with a blush of blood, probably due to gonioscopic lens compression.

Fig. 10-7

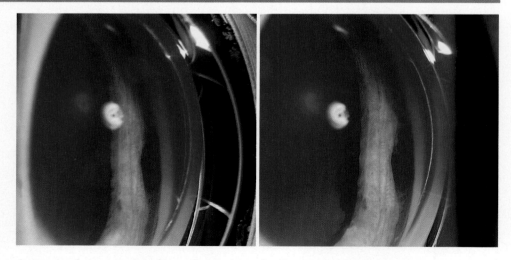

A goniophotograph of another ciliary body malignant melanoma extending forward into the angle. The tumor can be seen on both sides of the dilated iris.

Fig. 10-8

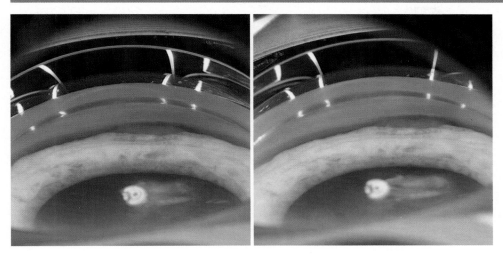

Ciliary body malignant melanoma that has caused local cataract formation, with an extension of amelanotic tumor tissue into the angle.

Fig. 10-9

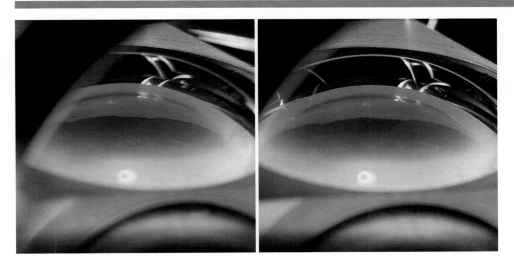

Ciliary body melanoma with extension into the angle to the right and evidence of tumor necrosis with heavy pigment extension into the angle on the left, representing melanomalytic glaucoma.

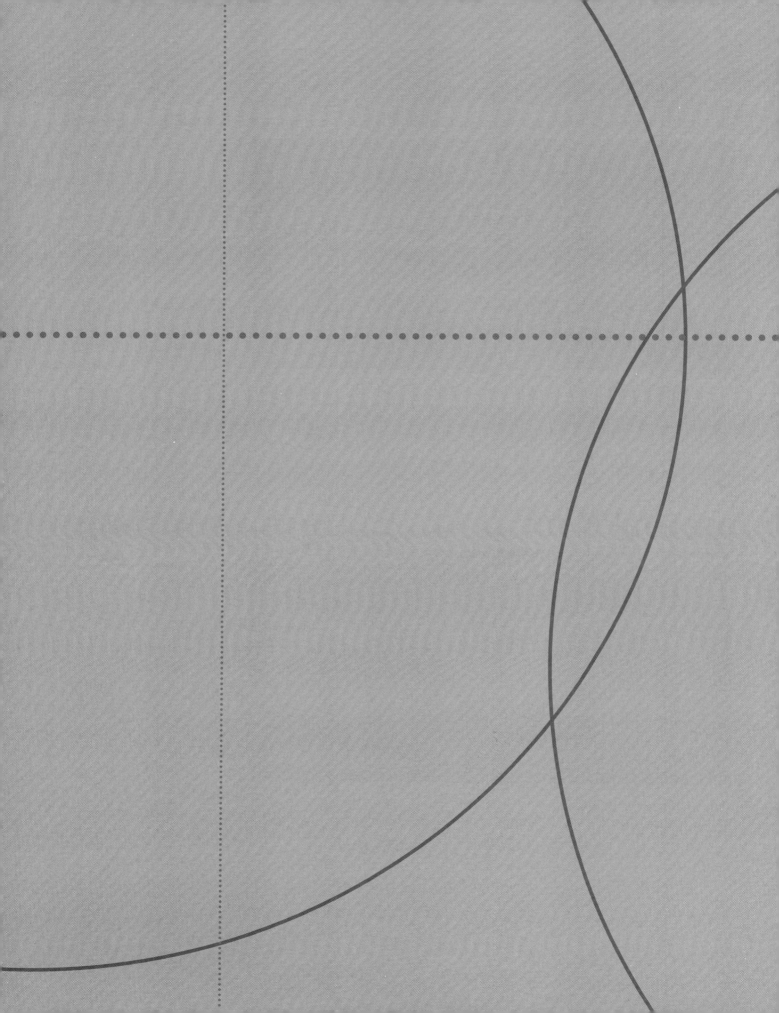

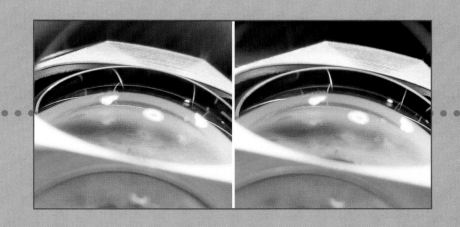

NEOVASCULAR GLAUCOMA

Neovascular glaucoma is a glaucoma secondary to the growth of vessels onto the trabecular meshwork accompanied by a fibrous membrane. This fibrovascular membrane can cover and obstruct outflow itself, or, more commonly, it can contract and pull the peripheral iris forward, causing complete synechial closure. The new vessel growth occurs primarily as a response to retinal ischemia. Neovascularization generally is first seen at the pupillary margin. It is very rare to see new vessel growth in other areas of the anterior segment in the absence of growth at the pupillary margin.

SUGGESTED READINGS

Alward WLM: Color atlas of gonioscopy, London, England, 1994, Wolfe Publishing (Mosby-Year Book Europe Limited), pp. 78–79.

Central Vein Occlusion Study Group: The Central Vein Occlusion Study, baseline and early natural history report, Arch Ophthalmol 111:1087, 1993.

Central Vein Occlusion Study Group: A randomized clinical trial of early panretinal photocoagulation for ischemic central retinal vein occlusion. Ophthalmology 102:1434, 1995.

Diabetic Retinopathy Study Research Group: Preliminary report on the effects of photocoagulation therapy. Am J Ophthalmol 81:383, 1976.

Diabetic Retinopathy Study Research Group: Four risk factors for severe visual loss in diabetic retinopathy. Arch Ophthalmol 97:654, 1979.

Dueker DK: Neovascular glaucoma. In Epstein DL, Allingham RR, and Schuman JS, editors: Chandler and Grant's glaucoma, ed 4, Baltimore, 1997, Williams & Wilkins, pp 366–371.

Hoskins HD Jr and Kass MA: Angle closure glaucoma without pupillary block. In Becker-Shaffer's diagnosis and therapy of the glaucomas, ed 6, St. Louis, 1989, Mosby-Year Book, Inc, pp 242–248.

Molteno ACB, Von Rooyen MMB, and Bartholomew RS: Implants for draining neovascular glaucoma. Br J Ophthalmol 61:120, 1977.

Simmons RJ et al: Goniophotocoagulation for neovascular glaucoma. Trans Am Acad Ophthalmol Otolaryngol 83:80, 1977.

Wand M: Neovascular glaucoma. In Ritch R, Shields MB, and Krupin T, editors: The glaucomas, ed 2, St. Louis, 1996, Mosby-Year Book, Inc, pp 1131–1139.

Wand M et al: Effects of panretinal photocoagulation on rubeosis iridis, angle neovascularization and neovascular glaucoma. Am J Ophthalmol 86:332, 1978.

Fig. 11-1

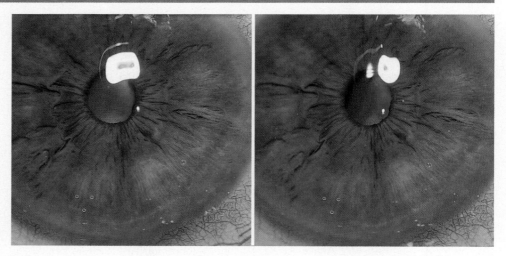

Anterior segment photograph of early anterior segment neovascularization showing fine neovascularization at the pupillary margin.

Fig. 11-2

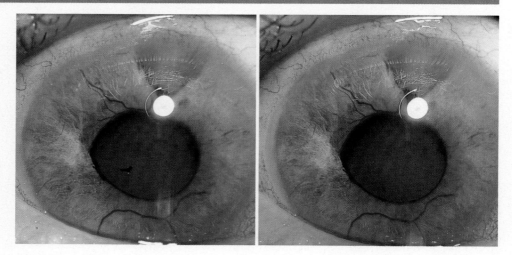

Anterior segment photograph of advanced neovascularization of the iris with secondary ectropion uveae and secondary iris dilation due to contraction within the fibrovascular membrane. A gray patch of iris atrophy due to prior high pressure can be seen at 9 o'clock. A surgical iridectomy exists superiorly.

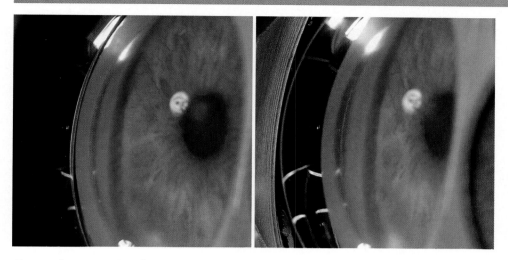

Fig. 11-3

Goniophotograph of extensive neovascularization of the iris and the angle. The trabecular meshwork is open but is covered entirely by new vessel growth.

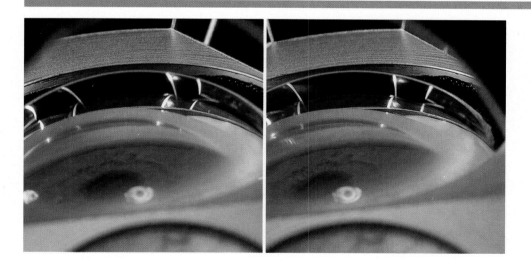

Fig. 11-4

Goniophotograph of an open angle covered by fine, threadlike neovascularization. The vessels do not extend beyond Schwalbe's line.

Fig. 11-5

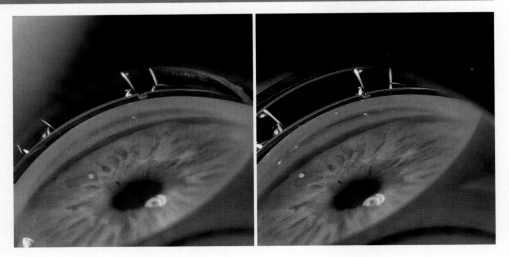

Goniophotograph of neovascularization of the trabecular meshwork with early peripheral anterior synechia formation to the right.

Fig. 11-6

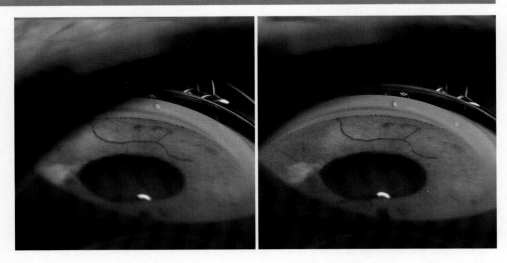

Goniophotograph of the inferior angle of a patient with neovascular glaucoma with complete synechial closure to the level of Schwalbe's line.

Fig. 11-7

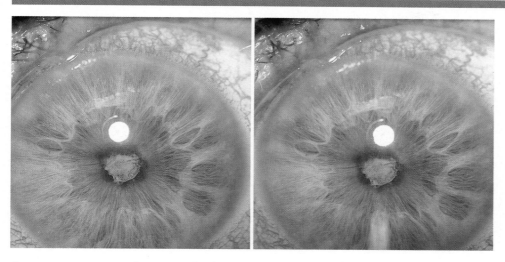

Anterior segment photograph showing extension of the fibrovascular membrane onto a cataractous lens with complete pupillary block and secondary iris bombé.

Fig. 11-8

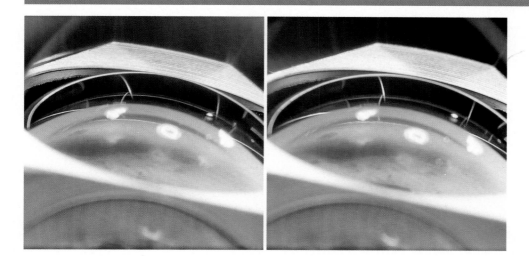

Occasionally a surgical wound, either a cataract incision or a filtration opening, will develop a fine neovascularization that causes easy bleeding (Swan syndrome). Goniophotograph of the neovascularization of a cataract incision, visible as a fine, reddish line within the trabecular meshwork, seen best above the peripheral iridectomy to the left.

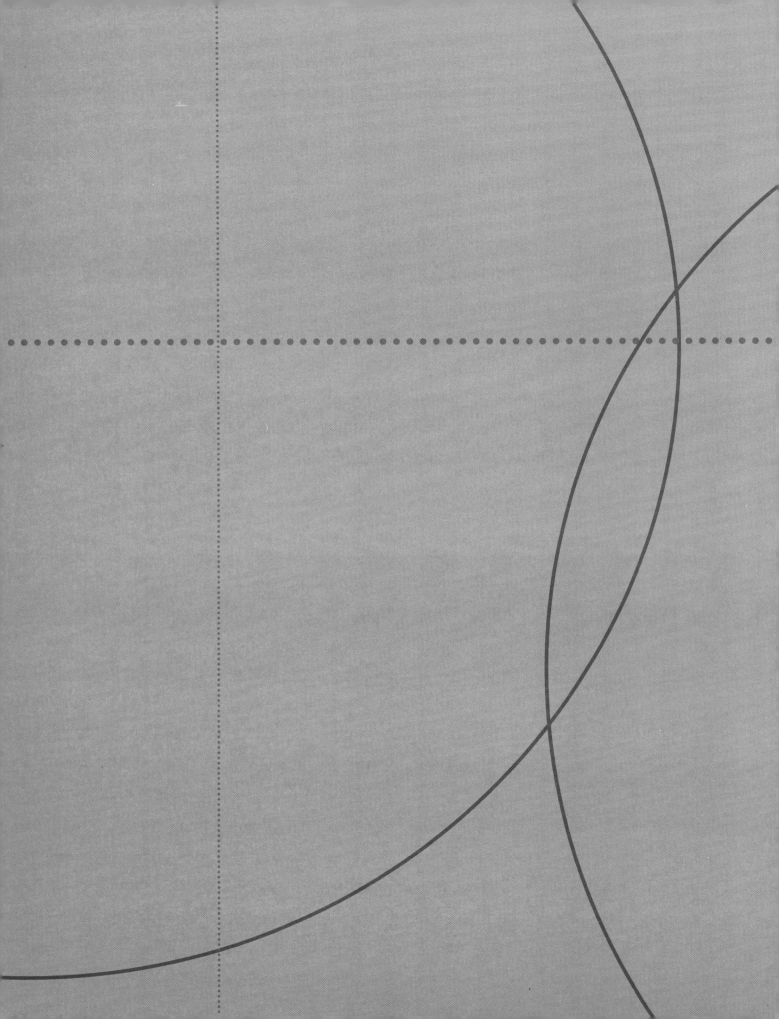

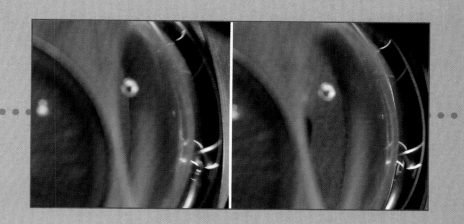

CHAPTER 12
CONGENITAL GLAUCOMA

In primary congenital glaucoma, the angle and outflow channels do not form normally, causing abnormal elevation of intraocular pressure. This abnormal elevation causes corneal enlargement, often with breaks in Descemet's membrane, called Haab's striae. The angle often reveals peripheral iris thinning, a high insertion of the iris, often approximately at the level of the scleral spur, and an indistinctness of the natural landmarks.

SUGGESTED READINGS

Allen L and Burian HM: Trabeculotomy ab externo. Am J Ophthalmol 53:19, 1962.

Allen L, Burian HM, and Braley AE: A new concept of the development of the anterior chamber angle. Arch Ophthalmol 53:783, 1955.

Alward WLM: Color atlas of gonioscopy, London, England, 1994, Wolfe Publishing (Mosby-Year Book Europe Limited), pp 57–59.

Barkan O: Technique of goniotomy. Arch Ophthalmol 19:217, 1938.

Buckley EG: Primary congenital open angle glaucoma. In Epstein DL, Allingham RR, and Schuman JS, editors: Chandler and Grant's glaucoma, ed 4, Baltimore, 1997, Williams & Wilkins, pp 598–608.

Dickens CJ and Hoskins HD Jr: Congenital glaucoma. In Ritch R, Shields MB, and Krupin T, editors: The glaucomas, ed 2, St. Louis, 1996, Mosby-Year Book, Inc, pp 729–749.

Freedman SF and Walton DS: Approach to infants and children with glaucoma. In Epstein DL, Allingham RR, and Schuman JS, editors: Chandler and Grant's glaucoma, ed 4, Baltimore, 1997, Williams & Wilkins, pp 586–597.

Hoskins HD Jr and Kass MA: Developmental and childhood glaucoma. In Becker-Shaffer's diagnosis and therapy of the glaucomas, ed 6, St. Louis, 1989, Mosby-Year Book, Inc, pp 355–381.

Hoskins HD Jr, Shaffer RN, and Hetherington J Jr: Anatomical classification of the developmental glaucomas. Arch Ophthalmol 102:1331, 1984.

Hoskins HD, Shaffer RN, and Hetherington J Jr: Goniotomy vs trabeculotomy. J Pediatric Ophthalmol Strab 21:153, 1984.

McPherson SD and Berry DP: Goniotomy vs external trabeculotomy for developmental glaucoma. Am J Ophthalmol 95:427, 1983.

Shaffer RN and Weiss DI: Congenital and pediatric glaucomas, St. Louis, 1970, Mosby.

Walton DS: Primary congenital open angle glaucoma: a study of the anterior segment abnormalities. Trans Am Ophthalmol Soc 77:746, 1979.

Worst JGF: Congenital glaucoma. Invest Ophthalmol 7:127, 1968.

Fig. 12-1

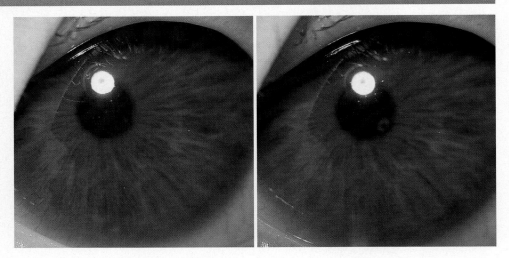

Anterior segment photograph of a patient with primary congenital glaucoma demonstrating an enlarged but clear cornea without Haab's striae.

Fig. 12-2

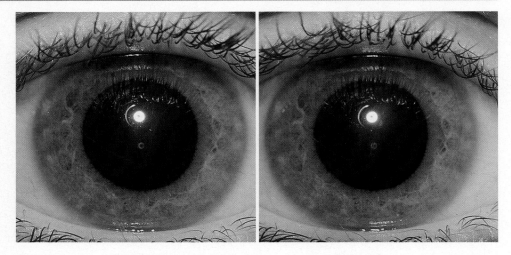

Anterior segment photograph of a patient with primary congenital glaucoma with an enlarged, clear cornea. A U-shaped Haab's striae extends from 9 o'clock up to 1 o'clock. The slightly rolled edges of the original break parallel each other.

Fig. 12-3

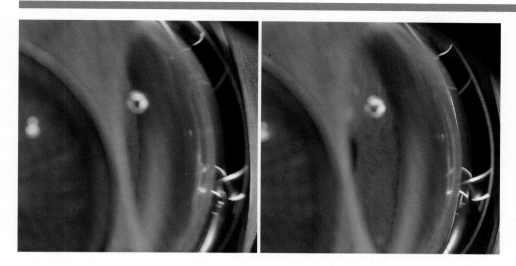

Goniophotograph of a young patient with primary congenital glaucoma revealing a flat iris with peripheral thinning and peripheral radial vessels. A high insertion to the level of the scleral spur is not visible above but is visible below. The trabecular meshwork is slightly grayish, and there is no definition to Schwalbe's line. There is no pigmentation within the trabecular meshwork, which is normal for the young.

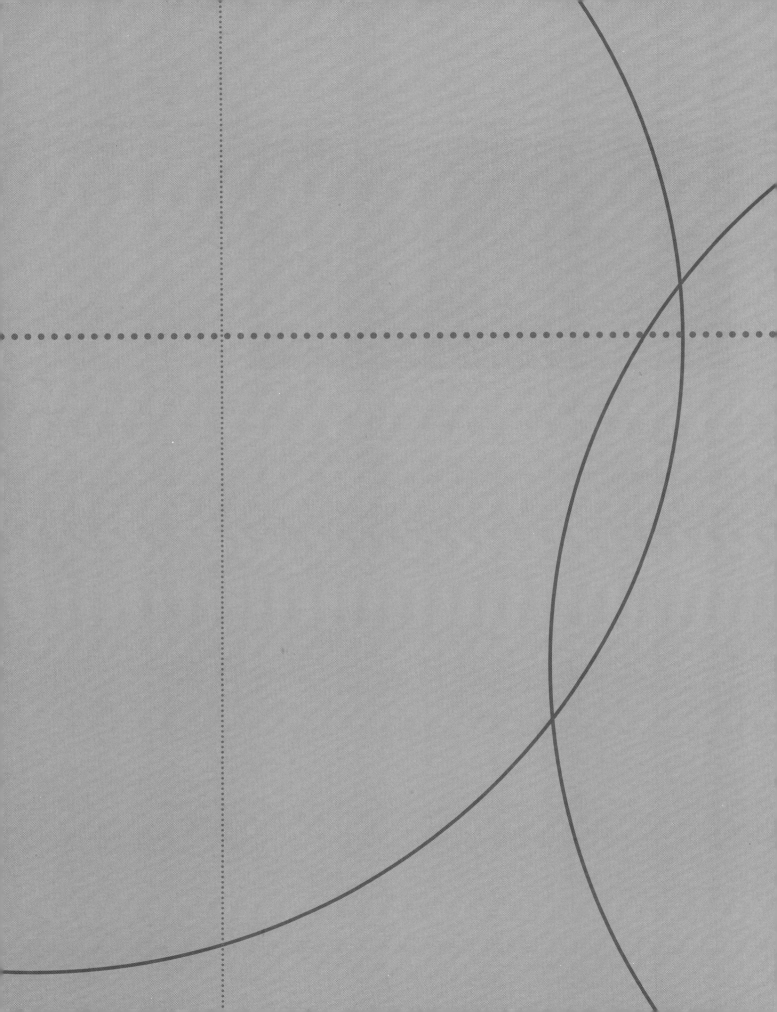

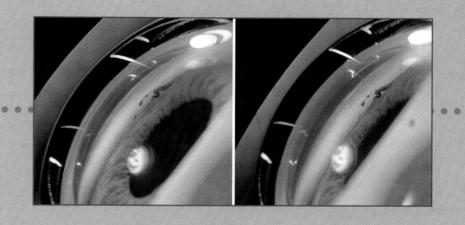

CHAPTER 13

ANTERIOR SEGMENT
DYSGENESIS

In anterior segment dysgenesis, the angle is malformed during development. Gonioscopic findings can vary from a prominent Schwalbe's ring (sometimes centrally displaced and called a posterior embryotoxon), to a finding of peripheral iris strands adhering to a permanent Schwalbe's ring, to Rieger syndrome. Rieger syndrome is characterized by posterior embryotoxon and peripheral iris adhesions associated with iris hypoplasia, often pupillary displacement, and glaucoma.

SUGGESTED READINGS

Axenfeld T: Embryotoxin corneae posterius. Ber Deutsch Ophth Ges 42:301, 1920.

Heon E et al: Linkage of autosomal dominant iris hypoplasia to the region of the Rieger syndrome locus (4q25). Hum Molec Genet 4:1435, 1995.

Hoskins HD Jr and Shaffer RN: Riegers syndrome: a form of irido-corneal mesodermal dysgenesis. Ped J Ophthalmol 9:26, 1972.

Mears AJ et al: Autosomal dominant iridogoniodysgenesis anomaly maps to 6p25. Am J Hum Genet 59:1321, 1996.

Mitchell JA et al: Deletions of different segments of the long arm of chromosome 4. Am J Med Genet 89:73, 1981.

Murray JC et al: Linkage of Rieger syndrome to the region of the epidermal growth factor gene on chromosome 4. Nature Genet 2:46, 1992.

Phillips JC et al: A second locus for Rieger syndrome maps to chromosome 13q14. Am J Hum Genet 59:613, 1996.

Rieger H: Dysgenesis mesodermalis corneae at iridis. Z Augenheilkd 86:333, 1935.

Shields MB: Axenfeld-Rieger syndrome: a theory of mechanism and distinctions from the iridocorneal endothelial syndrome. Trans Am Ophthalmol Soc 81:736, 1983.

Shields MB: Axenfeld-Rieger syndrome. In Ritch R, Shields MB, and Krupin T, editors: The glaucomas, ed 2, St. Louis, 1996, Mosby-Year Book, Inc, pp 875–885.

Shields MB et al: Axenfeld-Rieger syndrome: a spectrum of developmental disorders. Surv Ophthalmol 29:387, 1985.

Vaux C et al: Evidence the Rieger syndrome mapt to 4q25 or 4q27. J Med Genet 29:256, 1992.

Walton DS: Unusual pediatric glaucomas. In Epstein DL, Allingham RR, and Schuman JS, editors: Chandler and Grant's glaucoma, ed 4, Baltimore, 1997, Williams & Wilkins, pp 625–627.

Fig. 13-1

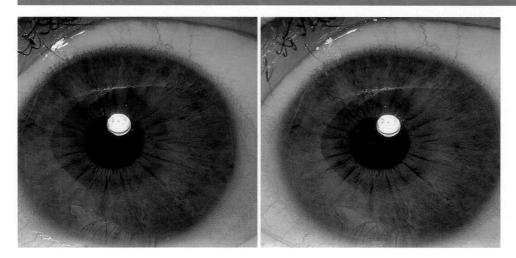

Anterior segment photograph of a patient with a prominent Schwalbe's ring, slightly displaced anteriorly, known as posterior embryotoxon.

Fig. 13-2

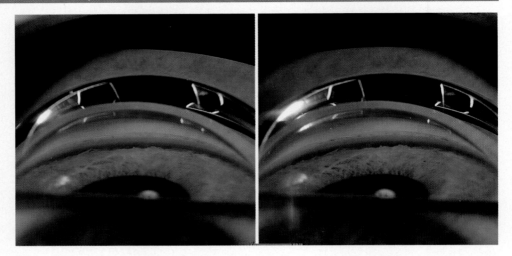

Goniophotograph of another patient with posterior embryotoxon. The rest of the angle appears grossly normal but without a delineated scleral spur.

Fig. 13-3

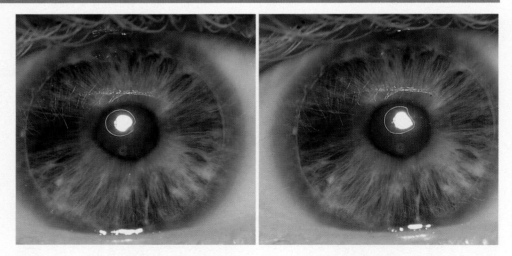

Anterior segment photograph of a patient with Axenfeld's anomaly showing a prominent, centrally displaced Schwalbe's ring with peripheral iris attachments. There is iris hypoplasia with loss of iris stroma.

Fig. 13-4

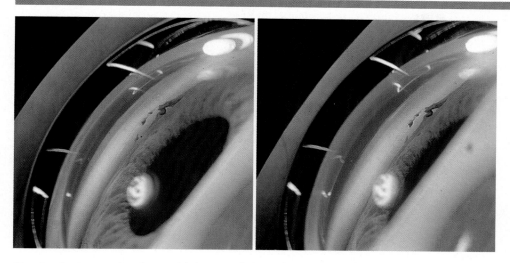

Goniophotograph of a mild form of Axenfeld's anomaly with peripheral iris strands adhering to a prominent Schwalbe's ring.

Fig. 13-5

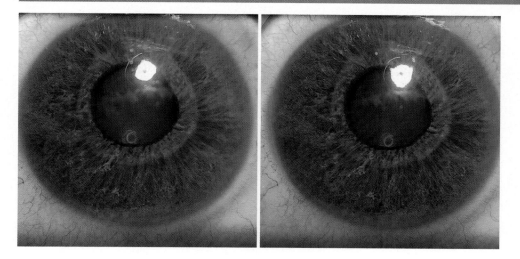

Anterior segment photograph of a patient with Rieger syndrome with severe iris hypoplasia, slight corectopia, angle anomalies, and glaucoma.

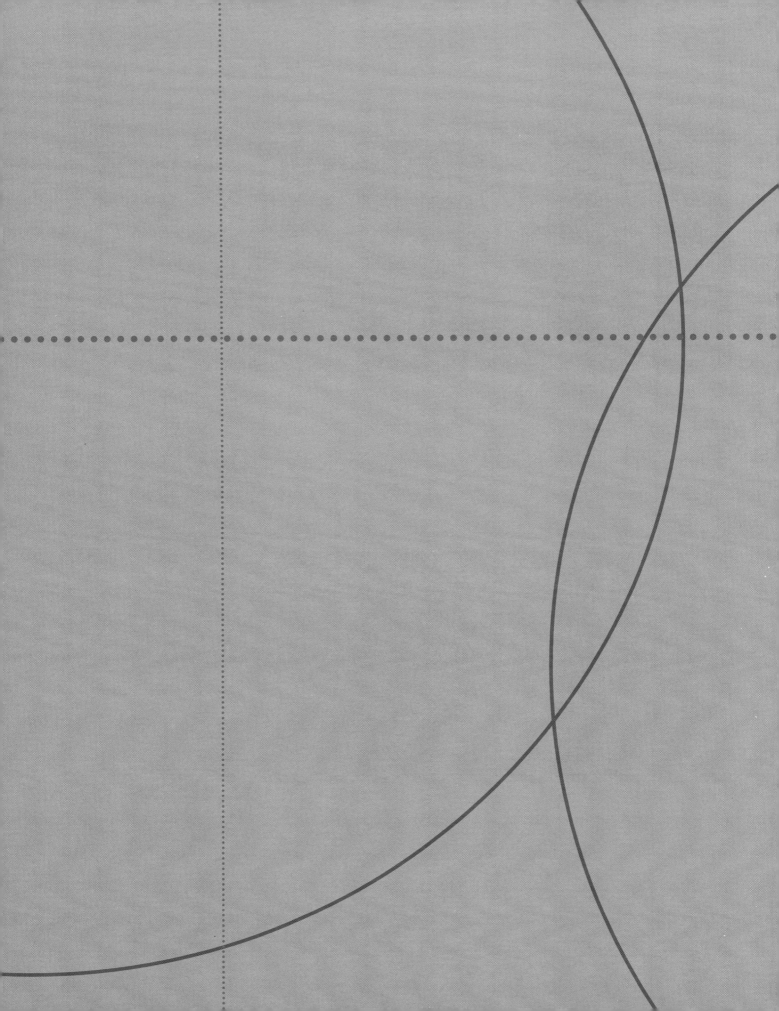

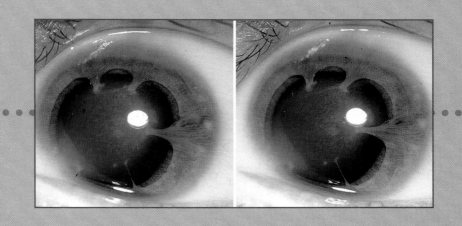

CHAPTER 14

MISCELLANEOUS CONDITIONS

Various conditions associated with glaucoma that do not warrant separate chapters are presented in this chapter.

SUGGESTED READINGS

Allen L, Burian HM, and Braley AE: A new concept of the development of the anterior chamber angle. Arch Ophthalmol 53:783, 1955.

Alward WLM: Color atlas of gonioscopy. London, England, 1994, Wolfe Publishing (Mosby-Year Book Europe Limited), pp 64–66.

Bahn CR et al: Classification of corneal endothelial disorders based on neural crest origin. Ophthalmology 91:558, 1984.

Bateman JB, Maumenee IH, and Sparkes RS: Peters' anomaly associated with partial deletion of the long arm of chromosome 2. Am J Ophthalmol 97:11, 1984.

Glaser T et al: PAX6 gene mutations in aniridia. In Wiggs JL, editor: Molecular genetics of ocular disease, New York, 1994, John Wiley & Sons, Inc, pp 83–98.

Hoskins HD Jr and Kass MA: Developmental and childhood glaucoma. In Becker-Shaffer's diagnosis and therapy of the glaucomas, ed 6, St. Louis, 1989, Mosby-Year Book, Inc, pp 382–391, 394–396.

Iwach AG et al: Analysis of surgical and medical management of glaucoma in Sturge-Weber syndrome. Ophthalmology 97:904, 1990.

Kupfer C, Kuwabara AT, and Stark WJ: The histopathology of Peters' anomaly. Am J Ophthalmol 80:653, 1975.

Mattox C: Glaucoma in the phakomatoses. In Epstein DL, Allingham RR, and Schuman JS, editors: Chandler and Grant's glaucoma, ed 4, Baltimore, 1997, Williams & Wilkins, pp 433–443.

Phelps CD: The pathogenesis of glaucoma in Sturge-Weber syndrome. Ophthalmology 85:276, 1978.

Reese AM and Ellsworth RM: The anterior chamber cleavage syndrome. Arch Ophthalmol 75:307, 1966.

Schottenstein EM: Petes' Anomaly. In Ritch R, Shields MB, and Krupin T, editors: The glaucomas, ed 2, St. Louis, 1996, Mosby-Year Book, Inc, pp 887–897.

Shingleton BJ: Glaucoma due to trauma. In Epstein DL, Allingham RR, and Schuman JS, editors: Chandler and Grant's glaucoma, ed 4, Baltimore, 1997, Williams & Wilkins, pp 401–402.

Teekhasaenee C et al: Glaucoma in oculodermal melanocytosis. Ophthalmology 97:562, 1990.

Walton DS: Unusual pediatric glaucomas. In Epstein DL, Allingham RR, and Schuman JS, editors: Chandler and Grant's glaucoma, ed 4, Baltimore, 1997, Williams & Wilkins, pp 629–631.

Weiss DI and Krohn DL: Benign melanocytic glaucoma complicating oculodermal melanocytosis. Ann Ophthalmol 3:958, 1971.

Fig. 14-1

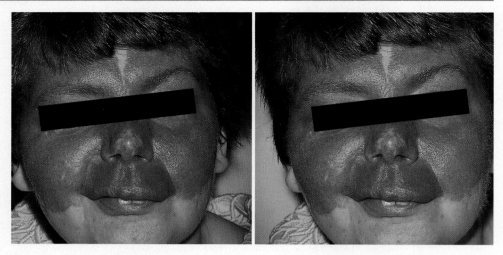

Encephalotrigeminal angiomatosis (Sturge–Weber disease). A patient showing bilateral facial involvement with bilateral hemangiomatosis of the conjunctiva, which can be associated with glaucoma.

Fig. 14-2

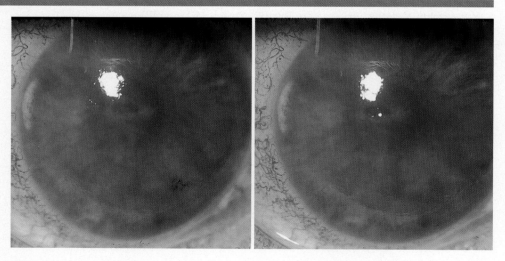

Glaucoma and secondary corneal edema due to Sturge–Weber disease.
Hemangiomatosis of the conjunctival vessels is visible.

Fig. 14-3

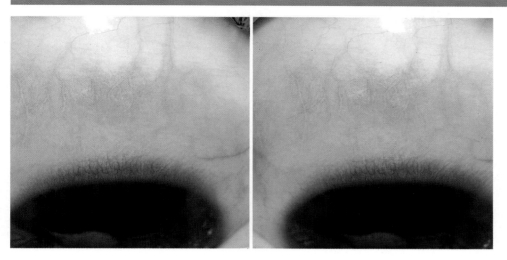

A patient with scleral melanocytosis. This patient also had lid involvement (oculodermal melanocytosis, known as nevus of Ota).

Fig. 14-4

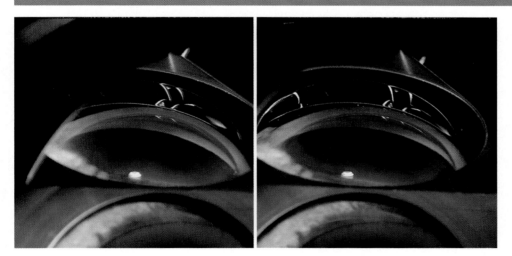

Goniophotograph of a patient with oculodermal melanocytosis and glaucoma, showing hyperpigmentation of the iris and angle.

Fig. 14-5

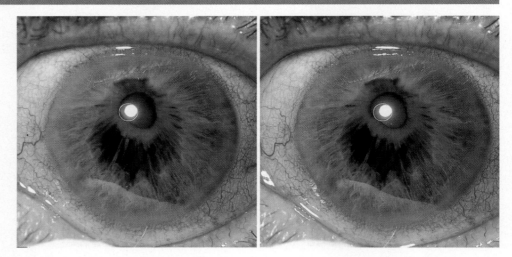

Iridoschisis. Anterior segment photograph of a patient with iridoschisis, a rare condition of the elderly, involving a splitting and separation of iris stromal fibers. The condition is relatively benign, bilateral, and should not be confused with the ICE syndrome.

Fig. 14-6

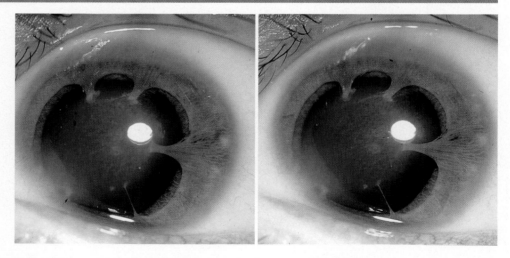

Peters' anomaly. Anterior segment photograph showing the characteristic central corneal opacity with posterior adhesions to the collarette region of the iris. An open-angle glaucoma, possibly due to angle maldevelopment, can be associated.

Fig. 14-7

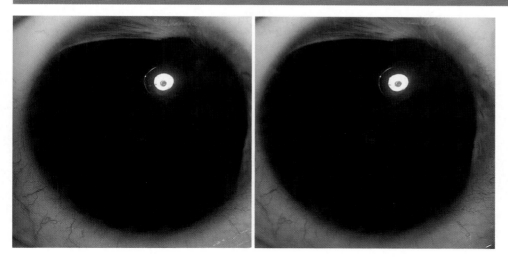

Aniridia. An anterior segment photograph showing almost complete absence of the iris, a portion of which can be seen superiorly and to the right. This hereditary, bilateral condition, with multiple ocular problems, can be associated with glaucoma.

Fig. 14-8

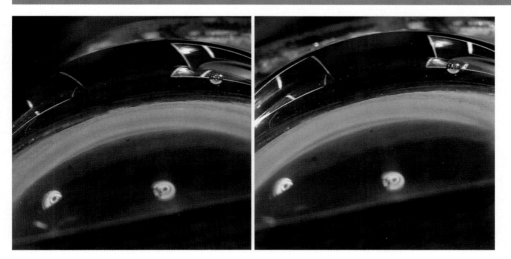

Goniophotograph of aniridia. A nubbin of iris tissue can be seen below the open angle. Later, the angle can be closed by this remnant of iris tissue.

Fig. 14-9

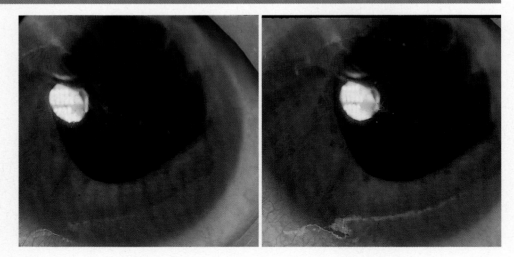

Epithelialization in the anterior chamber. This anterior segment photograph reveals an epithelial membrane descending down the endothelium from a superior cataract incision that was not closed fully. The undulating, beaded, heaped-up leading edge is pathognomonic for this condition, which can cause glaucoma.

Fig. 14-10

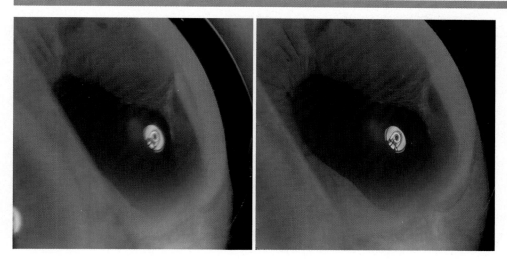

A grayish epithelial cyst in the angle.

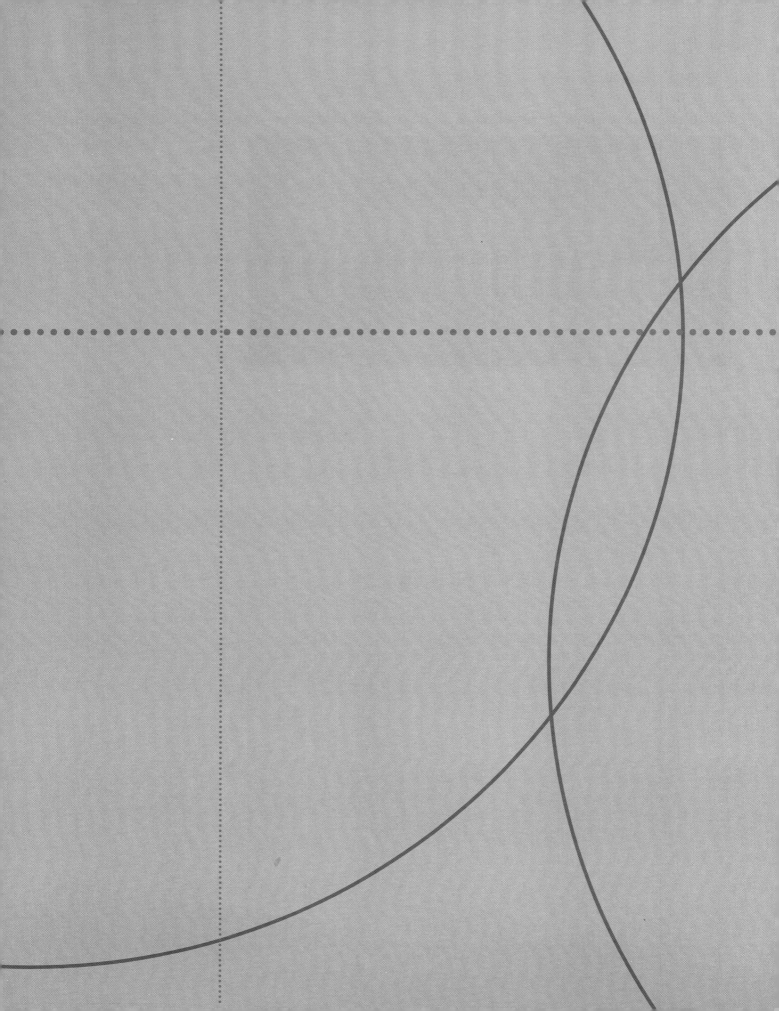

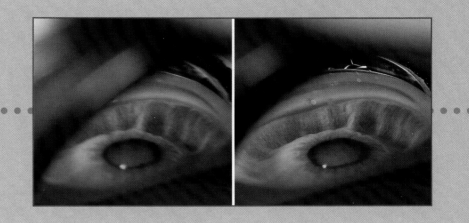

Abnormally decreased intraocular pressure can occur after filtration surgery, in association with a rhegmatogenous retinal detachment, after the creation of a cyclodialysis cleft (see Chapter 7), or in association with pharmacologically induced ocular hypotony, especially with the use of antiglaucoma medications after prior surgery.

SUGGESTED READINGS

Beigelman MN: Acute hypotony in retinal detachment. Arch Ophthalmol 1:463, 1929.

Campbell DG: Iris retraction syndrome associated with rhegmatogenous retinal detachment syndrome and hypotony: a new explanation. Arch Ophthalmol 102:1457, 1984.

Kawano S and Marmor MF: Metabolic influences on the absorption of serous subretinal fluid. Invest Ophthalmol Vis Sci 29:1255, 1988.

Nuyts RMMA et al: Treatment of hypotonous maculopathy after trabeculectomy and mitomycin-C. Am J Ophthalmol 118:322, 1994.

Pederson JE: Ocular hypotony. In Ritch R, Shields MB, and Krupin T, editors: The glaucomas, ed 2, St. Louis, 1996, Mosby-Year Book, Inc, pp 385–395.

Stampfer RL, McMenemy MG, and Lieberman MF: Hypotonous maculopathy after trabeculectomy with subconjunctival 5-fluorouracil. Am J Ophthalmol 114:544, 1992.

Van Heuven WAJ, Lam KW, and Ray GS: Source of subretinal fluid on the basis of ascorbate analyses. Arch Ophthalmol 100:976, 1982.

Vela MA and Campbell DG: Hypotony and ciliochoroidal detachment following pharmacologic aqueous suppressant therapy in previously filtered patients. Ophthalmology 92: 50, 1985.

Fig. 15-1

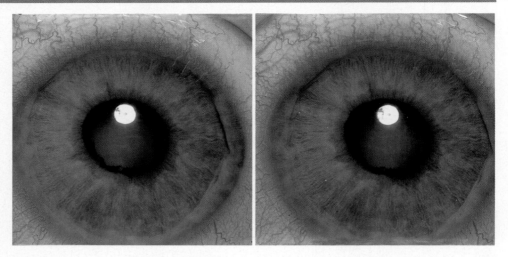

The iris retraction syndrome. Anterior segment photograph of a patient with a deepened anterior chamber and a peripheral iris that falls almost straight posterior. Pupillary synechiae to the lens are present. In this syndrome, a rhegmatogenous retinal detachment exists. When the subretinal fluid removal mechanism exceeds production, the lens and the iris are pulled posteriorly and the intraocular pressure decreases to almost zero.

Fig. 15-2

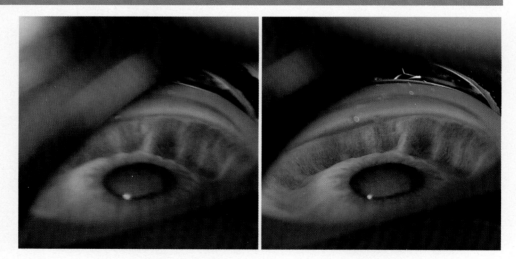

The iris retraction syndrome. Goniophotograph of another patient with hypotony and the iris retraction configuration. The angle is partially closed due to a preceding iris bombé configuration. Posterior synechias to a cataractous lens can be seen.

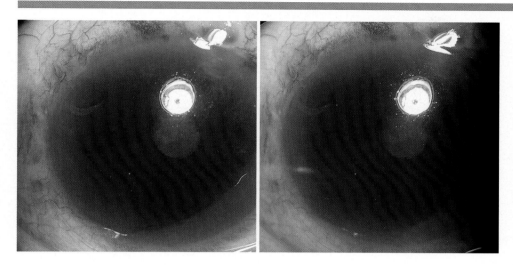

Pharmacologically induced ocular hypotony syndrome. Shallow anterior chamber and profound hypotony induced by topical beta-blocker use in a patient with a failed filtration operation, with large secondary choroidal effusions as well.

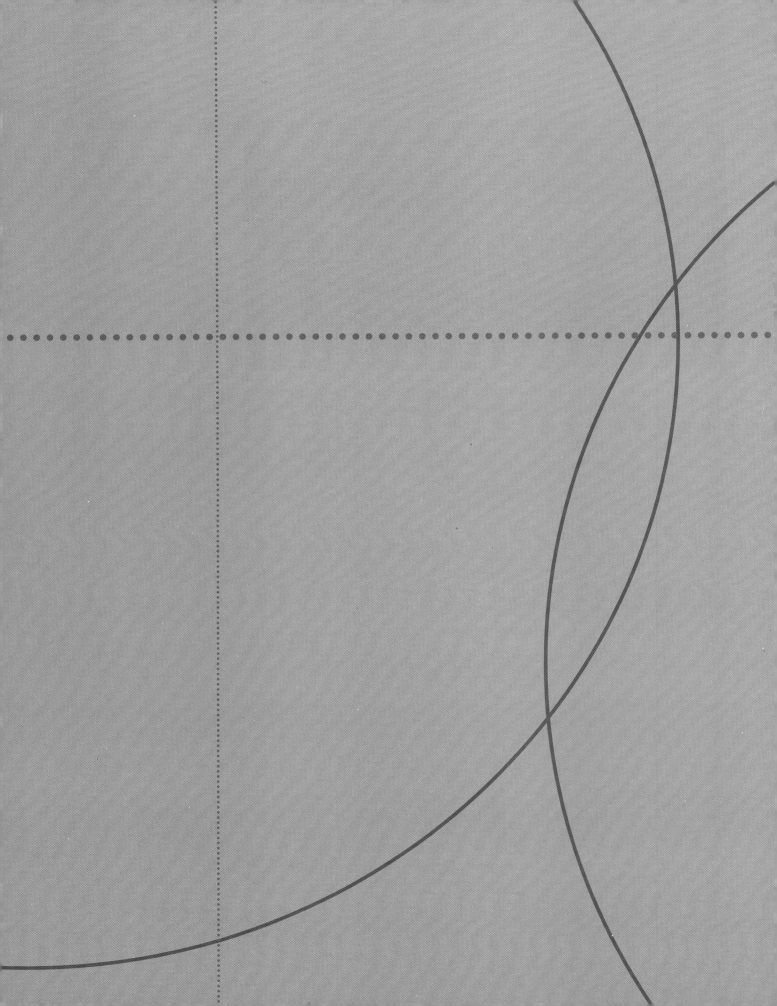

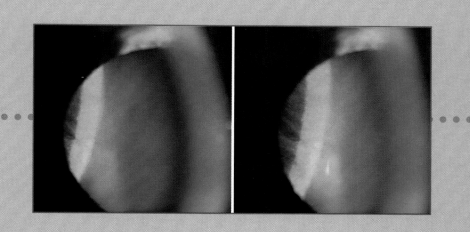

CHAPTER 16

SURGERY

Patients with intractable elevation of intraocular pressure may be treated with filtration surgery, which is intended to create a fistula to bypass the usual pathways for aqueous outflow from the eye. An opening, either guarded or unguarded, is made through the limbus into the anterior chamber, creating an external filtration bleb.

SUGGESTED READINGS

Allingham RR: Filtering surgery in the management of glaucoma. In Epstein DL, Allingham RR, and Schuman JS, editors: Chandler and Grant's glaucoma, ed 4, Baltimore, 1997, Williams & Wilkins, pp 516–537.

Bellows AR: Postoperative management following filtration surgery. In Epstein DL, Allingham RR, and Schuman JS, editors: Chandler and Grant's glaucoma, ed 4, Baltimore, 1997, Williams & Wilkins, 538–550.

Chen CW et al: Trabeculectomy with topical application of mitomycin-C in refractory glaucoma. J Ocul Pharmacol 6:175, 1990.

Fluorouracil Filtering Surgery Study Group: Three-year follow-up of the fluorouracil filtering surgery study. Am J Ophthalmol 115:82, 1993.

Hoskins HD Jr and Kass MA: Surgical techniques. In Becker-Shaffer's diagnosis and therapy of the glaucomas, ed 6, St. Louis, 1989, Mosby-Year Book, Inc, pp 542–637.

Katz LJ, Costa VP, and Spaeth GL: Filtration surgery. In Ritch R, Shields MB, and Krupin T, editors: The glaucomas, ed 2, St. Louis, 1996, Mosby-Year Book, Inc, pp 1661–1702.

Liebmann JM and Ritch R: Complications of glaucoma filtering surgery. In Ritch R, Shields MB, and Krupin T, editors: The glaucomas, ed 2, St. Louis, 1996, Mosby-Year Book, Inc, pp 1703–1736.

Parrish RK II and Folberg R: Wound healing in glaucoma surgery. In Ritch R, Shields MB, and Krupin T, editors: The glaucomas, ed 2, St. Louis, 1996, Mosby-Year Book, Inc, pp 1633–1651.

Skuta GL et al: Intraoperative mitomycin versus postoperative 5-fluorouracil in high-risk glaucoma filtering surgery. Ophthalmology 99:438, 1992.

Fig. 16-1

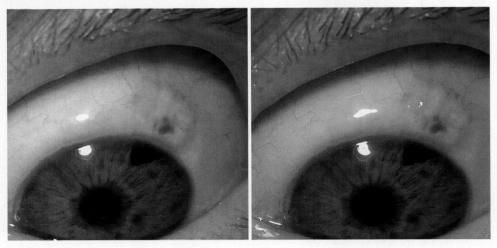

A filtration procedure (trephine) with an overlying, functioning filtration bleb.

Fig. 16-2

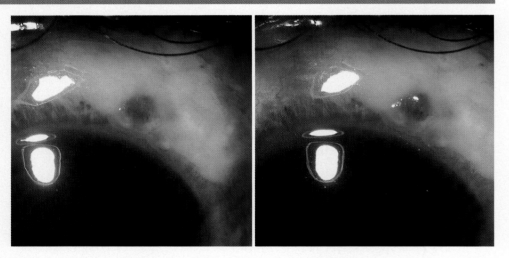

Another functioning filtration bleb over a full-thickness trephine opening.

Fig. 16-3

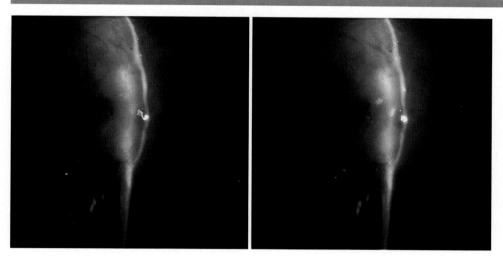

Slit-lamp view of the bleb shown in Fig. 16-2 showing fine microcysts in the conjunctiva, generally a sign of successful filtration.

Fig. 16-4

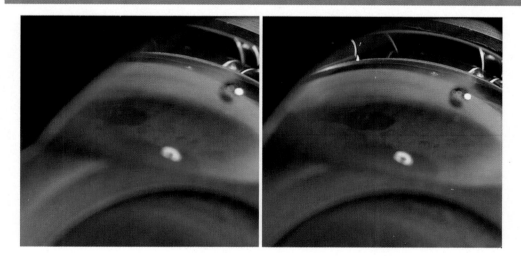

Gonioscopic view of patent internal opening for filtration positioned above the surgical iridectomy.

Fig. 16-5

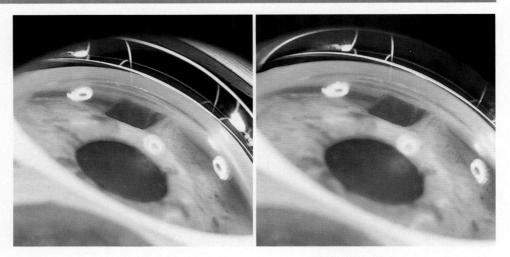

Goniophotograph showing internal blockage of a filtration procedure with iris, ciliary process, and fibrotic vitreous to the internal opening.

Fig. 16-6

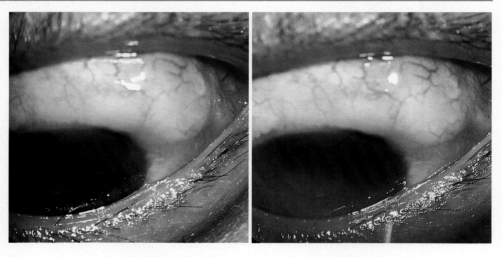

External view of a thick-walled (encapsulated), failed filtration bleb.

Fig. 16-7

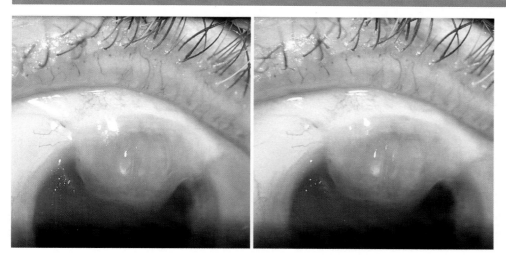

External view of a filtration bleb that has dissected down onto the cornea.

Fig. 16-8

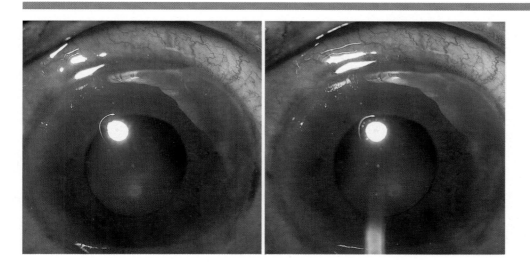

After filtration surgery and associated with hypotony, complications in the immediate postoperative period can include the development of a shallow anterior chamber.

Fig. 16-9

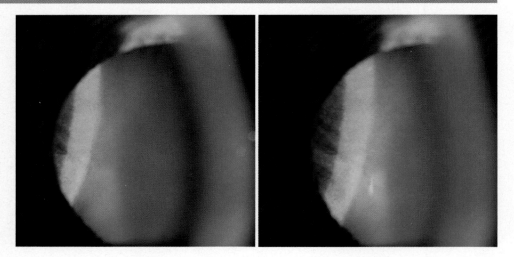

Postoperative development of secondary suprachoroidal effusions, seen behind the lens.

Fig. 16-10

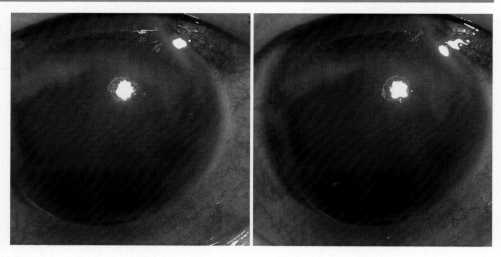

Postoperative hemorrhage, seen here both into the anterior chamber and into the bleb.

Fig. 16-11

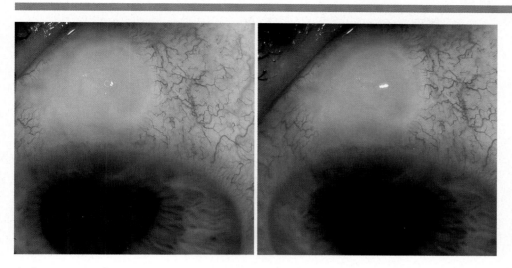

A later complication can occur with bleb infection that can progress to endophthalmitis. Seen here are the classic signs of early bleb infection, a pale, milky bleb surrounded by conjunctival hyperemia.

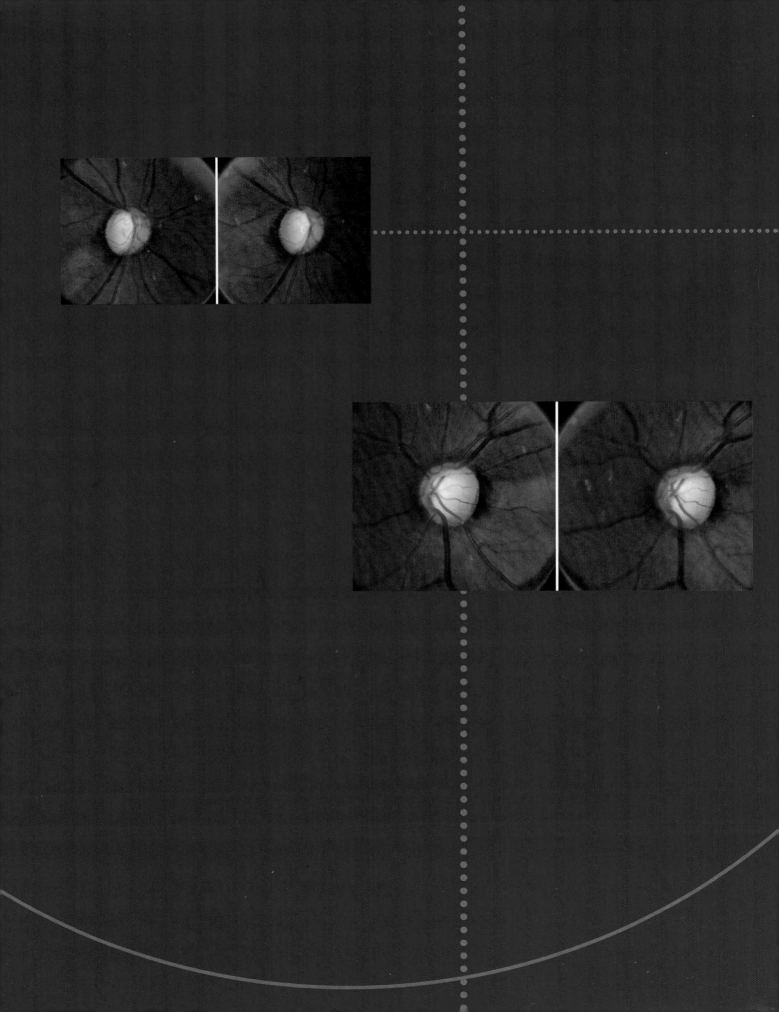

PART TWO

THE OPTIC NERVE

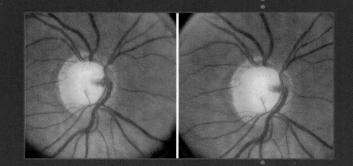

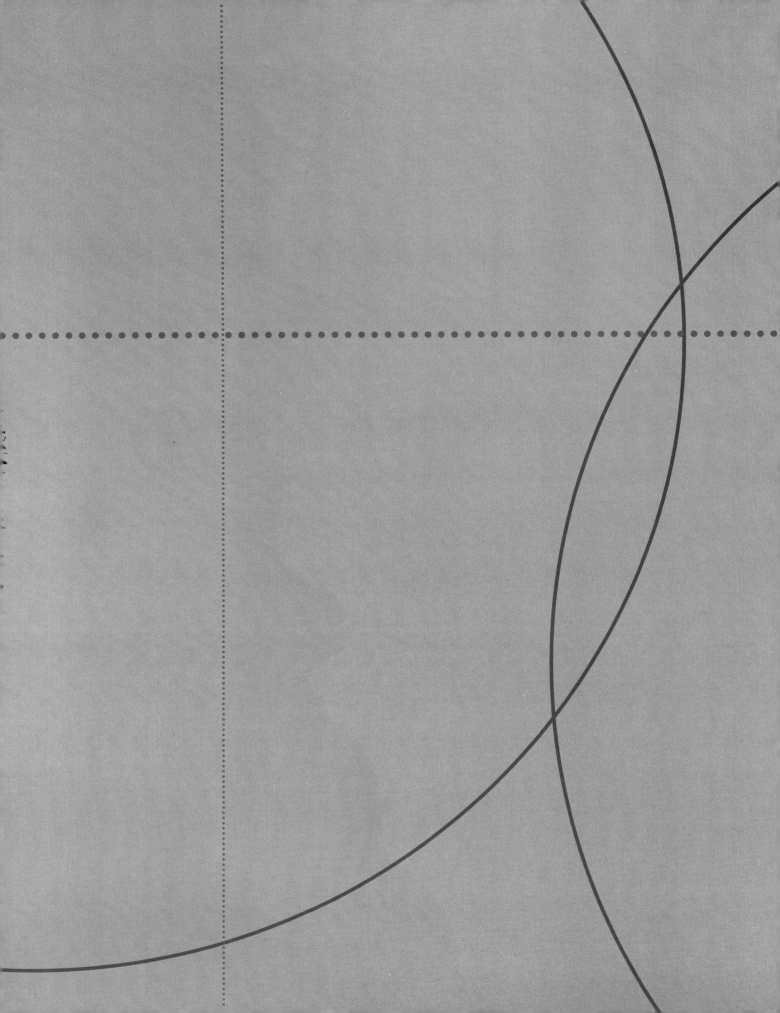

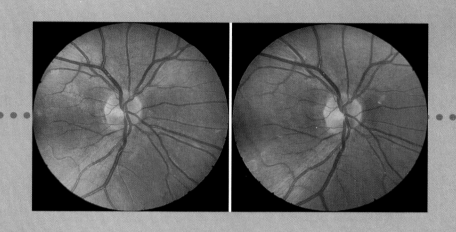

CHAPTER 17

NORMAL OPTIC NERVE
AND DOCUMENTATION OF
CLINICAL FINDINGS

Anatomy and Clinical Appearance

The optic nerve is composed of four parts: intraocular, intraorbital, intracanalicular, and intracranial.[1,2] The intracranial portion of the optic nerve joins with the contralateral optic nerve to form the optic chiasm. The optic tract is the neural connection between the optic chiasm and the lateral geniculate body, and the optic radiations project from the lateral geniculate nucleus to the visual cortex. The intraocular portion of the optic nerve, which is damaged in glaucoma, may be divided into four parts: the nerve fiber layer, and prelaminar, laminar, and postlaminar regions. The arterial blood supply of the anterior optic nerve is derived primarily from branches of the short posterior ciliary arteries, with few arterial connections between the choroid or the central retinal artery and this portion of the optic nerve.[3,4]

The prelaminar portion of the optic nerve is visible on clinical evaluation, varying in appearance between individuals (Figs. 17-1 – 17-3). The retinal ganglion cell axons exit the eye through the posterior scleral foramen. The internal surface of the posterior scleral opening is visible by clinical ophthalmoscopy as the optic nerve head or optic disc. The mean ± standard deviation area of the optic disc, based on a study of 571 normal eyes, was 2.69 ± 0.70 mm^2.[5] The optic disc is larger in highly myopic eyes and smaller in highly hyperopic eyes, compared with normal eyes. The area within the peripapillary scleral ring consists of the neural rim and the optic cup. In 571 normal eyes, the mean ± standard deviation cup area was 0.73 ± 0.59 mm^2.[5] The optic disc is slightly vertically oval, whereas the normal cup is slightly horizontally oval.

The peripapillary scleral ring of Elschnig is a white band surrounding the optic nerve head, which separates the intrapapillary area of the optic disc from the parapapillary area. This ring may be visualized more easily in eyes with optic nerve damage but also may be identified in normal eyes. On clinical examination, the ring may be broadest temporally, thinner superotemporally and inferotemporally, and narrowest nasally. Retinal nerve fibers pass over the scleral ring of Elschnig to within the optic nerve head to form the neural rim, which is the focus of clinical optic nerve evaluation.

The retinal nerve fiber layer can be visualized around the optic nerve head by clinical ophthalmoscopy and red-free, wide-angle fundus photographs as bright striations in the retinal reflex (Fig. 17-4). The axons of the ganglion cells nasal to the optic disc run directly toward the disc, whereas those from the temporal retina follow an arcuate course superior and inferior to the fovea.[5] The nerve fiber layer thickness is greatest superior and inferior to the optic disc and is least nasal and temporal to the disc. The retinal nerve fiber layer is composed primarily of ganglion cell axons and retinal vessels, admixed with some astrocytes and Müller cell processes. The basal lamina of the Müller cell processes forms the internal limiting membrane, which is the inner covering of the nerve fiber layer. With glaucomatous damage, vessels may lose their nerve fiber covering and become demarcated more clearly, and atrophic thinning or defects may become visible by careful clinical evaluation.

On histologic evaluation, the neural rim in the prelaminar region normally is composed of unmyelinated optic nerve fibers and a small proportion of astrocytes and glial processes. Occasionally, myelinated nerve fibers may be observed by clinical ophthalmoscopy (Fig. 17-5). With glaucomatous optic nerve atrophy, the laminar region may be apparent, particularly the pores or trabeculae that allow passage of axon bundles through the lamina cribrosa. The human lamina cribrosa has approximately 500 to 600 pores, which vary in size. The pore areas in the superior and inferior quadrants are significantly larger than those in the nasal and temporal quadrants.[1]

Documentation of Clinical Findings

One method used by clinicians to describe the appearance of the optic nerve head is estimation of the cup-to-disc ratio (Fig. 17-6). In normal eyes, variation exists in the cup-to-disc ratio. The cup-to-disc ratio usually is larger horizontally than vertically in normal eyes. Glaucomatous optic nerve damage is associated with vertical elongation of the cup or notching of the neural rim, which may affect estimates of the cup-to-disc ratio. Asymmetry of the cup-to-disc ratio is a helpful finding, because a difference of more than 0.2 in the horizontal cup-to-disc ratio was reported to occur in less than 1% of the normal population.[6] One example of asymmetry of cup and disc sizes in normal eyes of one individual is anisometropia. The cup-to-disc ratio may be described as an overall estimate, or may be divided into horizontal and vertical estimates.

Optic disc drawing is a convenient and inexpensive method for documenting the appearance of the optic nerve head.[7] This technique is especially useful when optic nerve photographs cannot be obtained, such as in patients with miotic pupils or significant media opacity. There are, however, limitations of this approach. Clinical interpretation of the appearance of the optic nerve head is subjective, and artistic methods for representing the findings may vary among observers.

The usual method for disc drawing represents the cup as an inner circle within a larger circle depicting the outer margin of the disc (Fig. 17-7). A well-defined, abrupt drop-off in the neural rim may be represented by a solid line, whereas areas of sloping or uncertainty may be shown with a hatched line. Other findings that may be drawn include abnormalities of blood vessels, optic disc hemorrhage, laminar pores, and peripapillary atrophy of the retinal pigment epithelium. Although en face drawings are shown more commonly, an estimation of the profile appearance of the optic nerve head may be drawn. Serial drawings can be used to document progressive optic disc cupping in glaucomatous eyes, and a 10-square grid may improve the accuracy of drawings of the cup dimensions.[8]

However, cup-to-disc ratios and optic nerve head drawings are imprecise and lack reproducibility.[9] A variety of cameras may be used to photograph the optic disc, although the results can be impaired by miotic pupils, media opacity, or poor patient cooperation. Photographs of the optic nerve head are superior to drawings and cup-to-disc ratio estimates because they contain a great deal of accurate information. Stereo fundus photographs may be taken sequentially or simultaneously, with a fixed angle between images. Simultaneous stereo photographs provide a standard, reproducible view of the optic nerve head with excellent stereopsis. The limitation of stereo photographs is not the information contained in the images but rather the subjective interpretation of this information by clinicians.[9] Because of this limitation, more quantitative, objective, and reproducible methods of optic nerve head analysis have been developed (Fig. 17-8). Computer-assisted analysis of optic nerve head topography has been described using digital processing of optic nerve head images, computed raster stereography, and laser scanners.[10,11]

REFERENCES

1. Varma R and Minckler DS: Anatomy and pathophysiology of the retina and optic nerve. In Ritch R, Shields MB, and Krupin T: The glaucomas, ed 2, Philadelphia, 1996, Mosby-Year Book, Inc, pp 139-175.

2. Hoskins HD and Kass M: Becker-Shaffer's diagnosis and therapy of the glaucomas, ed 6, Philadelphia, 1989, CV Mosby, pp 178-189.

3. Cioffi GA and Van Buskirk EM: Vasculature of the anterior optic nerve and peripapillary choroid. In Ritch R, Shields MB, and Krupin T: The glaucomas, ed 2, Philadelphia, 1996, Mosby-Year Book, Inc, pp 177-188.

4. Hayreh SS: Blood supply of the optic nerve head in health and disease. In Lambrou GN and Greve EL, editors: Ocular blood flow in glaucoma, Amsterdam, 1989, Kugler & Ghedini Publications, pp 3-48.

5. Jonas JB and Naumann GOH: The optic nerve: its embryology, histology, and morphology. In Varma R and Spaeth GL: The optic nerve in glaucoma, Philadelphia, 1993, J.B. Lippincott, pp 3-26.

6. Armaly MF: Optic cup in normal and glaucomatous eyes. Invest Ophthalmol 9:425, 1970.

7. Katz LJ: Optic disc drawings. In Varma R and Spaeth GL: The optic nerve in glaucoma, Philadelphia, 1993, J.B. Lippincott, pp 147-158.

8. Shaffer RN et al: The use of diagrams to record changes in glaucomatous disks. Am J Ophthalmol 80:460, 1975.

9. Lichter PR: Variability of expert observers in evaluating the optic disc. Trans Am Ophthalmol Soc 74:532, 1976.

10. Kalina PH, Hutchinson BT, and Netland PA: Quantitative assessment of optic nerve head topography. Int Ophthalmol Clin 34:239, 1994.

11. Schuman JS, editor: Imaging in glaucoma, Thorofare, NJ, 1997, Slack, Inc.

Fig. 17-1

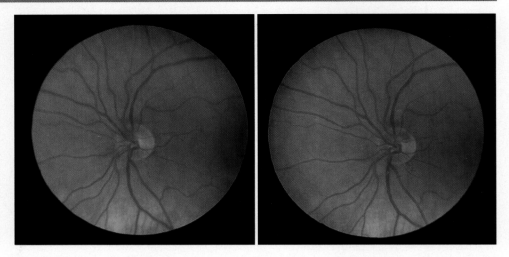

Normal left optic nerve head. The prelaminar portion of the optic nerve is visible on clinical evaluation. The neural rim is intact in this healthy individual and has a pink to reddish hue. There is a small optic cup.

Fig. 17-2

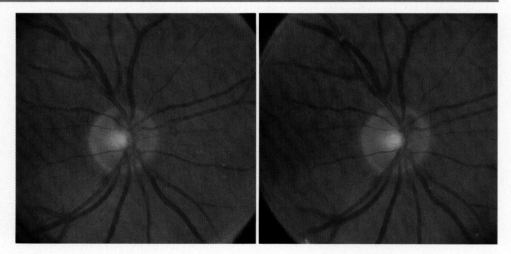

Higher magnification view of normal right optic nerve head. The area within the peripapillary scleral ring consists of the neural rim and the optic cup. The scleral ring of Elschnig is a white band surrounding the optic nerve head.

The appearance of the normal optic nerve head varies between individuals.

Fig. 17-3

Fig. 17-3A

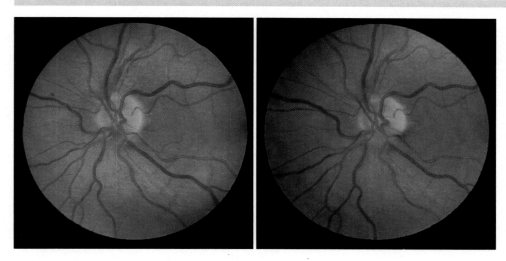

Normal-appearing left optic nerve head with a small optic cup.

Fig. 17-3B

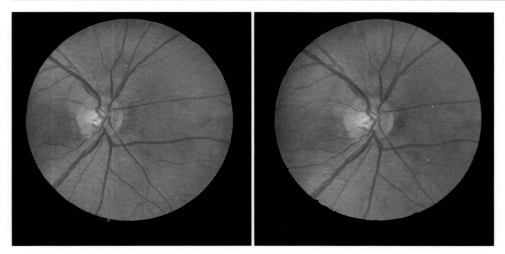

Right optic nerve head in a healthy individual with an intact neural rim and a larger optic cup compared with Fig. 17-3A.

Fig. 17-4
The retinal nerve fiber layer, which appears opthalmoscopically as bright striations in the retinal reflex. The axons nasal to the disc are directed toward the disc, whereas those from the temporal retina follow an arcuate course superior and inferior to the fovea. The nerve fiber layer is thicker superior and inferior to the disc compared with the nasal and temporal regions. Atrophy and defects in the nerve fiber layer may appear in glaucomatous eyes.

Fig. 17-4A

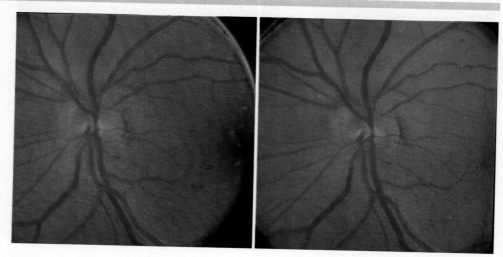

Example of normal left optic nerve head with visible striations in the retinal reflex in the peripapillary region due to the nerve fiber layer.

Fig. 17-4B

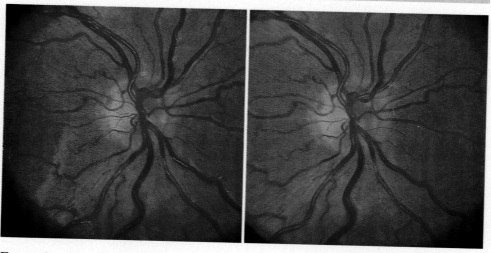

Example of normal right optic nerve head with visible striations in the retinal reflex in the peripapillary region due to the nerve fiber layer.

Myelinated nerve fibers. Myelination of nerve fibers around the optic nerve head varies in location and extent. They may be adjacent to or separate from the optic nerve head.

Fig. 17-5

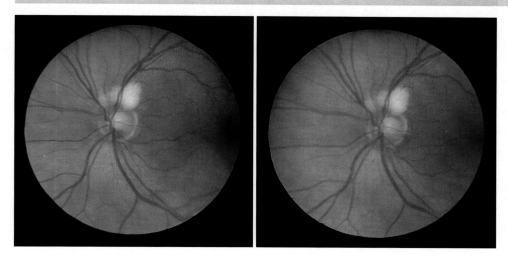

Fig. 17-5A

This example shows the left optic nerve head with myelination of nerve fibers located superiorly and contiguous with the disc.

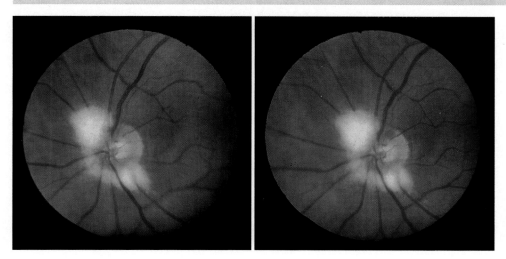

Fig. 17-5B

Left optic nerve head with myelination of nerve fibers contiguous with the disc, located on the nasal and inferior sides of the disc.

Fig. 17-5C

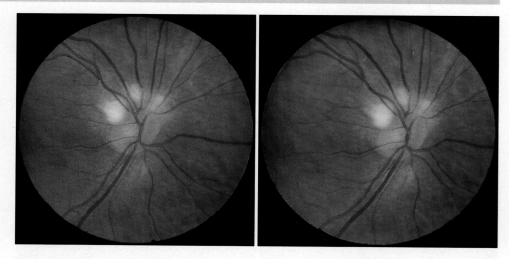

Varying degrees of myelination of nerve fibers in the right eye of the same individual as shown in Fig. 17-5D.

Fig. 17-5D

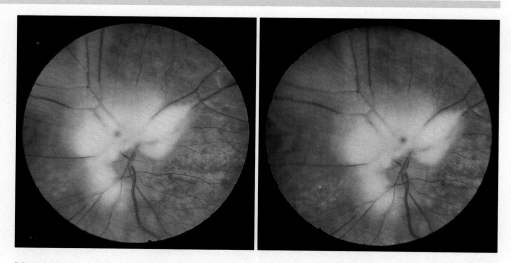

Varying degrees of myelination of nerve fibers in the left eye of the same individual as shown in Fig. 17-5C. There is more extensive myelination of nerve fibers in this left eye compared with the right eye shown in Fig. 17-5C.

Fig. 17-5E

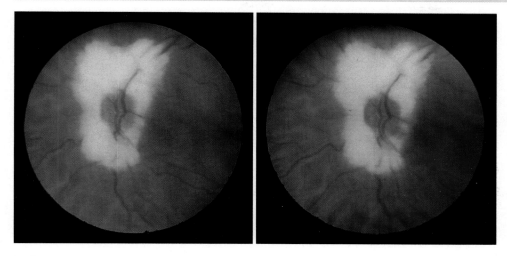

Left optic nerve head with myelination of nerve fibers surrounding the disc.

Fig. 17-6

Cup-to-disc ratio. The ratio of cup area to the disc area, or the ratio of the horizontal or vertical cup width to the disc width, may be estimated. The cup-to-disc ratio often is larger horizontally than vertically in normal eyes. The right optic discs in these examples demonstrate increasing cup-to-disc ratios.

Fig. 17-6A

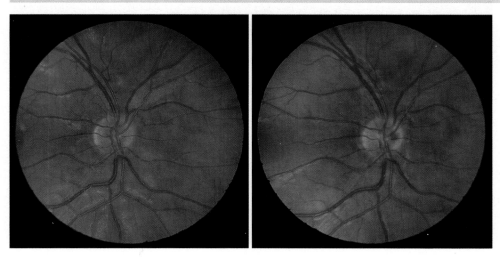

This example shows the right optic nerve head with no apparent cup (cup-to-disc ratio of 0).

Fig. 17-6B

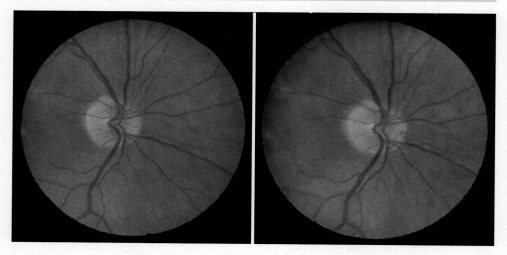

Right optic nerve head with cup-to-disc ratio of approximately 0.1.

Fig. 17-6C

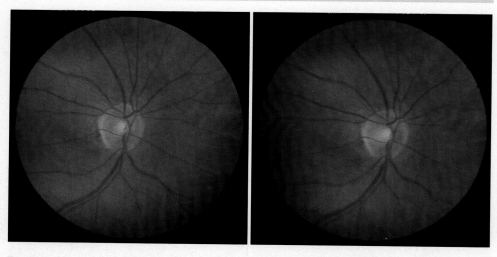

Right optic nerve head with cup-to-disc ratio of approximately 0.2.

Fig. 17-6D

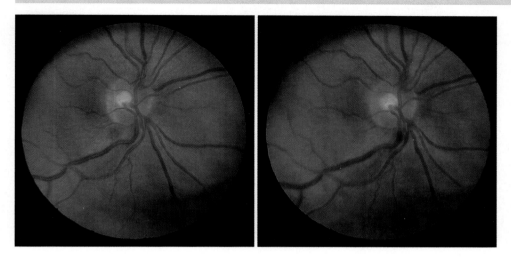

Right optic nerve head with cup-to-disc ratio of approximately 0.3.

Fig. 17-6E

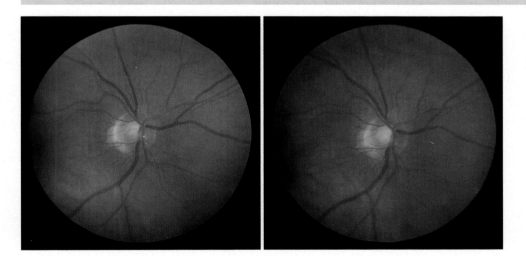

Right optic nerve head with cup-to-disc ratio of approximately 0.4.

Fig. 17-6F

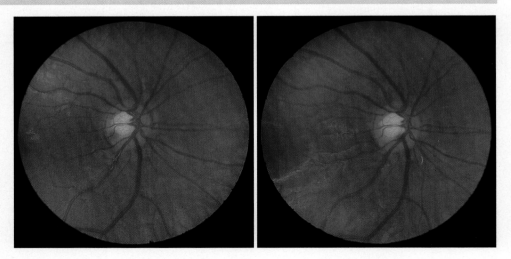

Right optic nerve head with cup-to-disc ratio of approximately 0.5.

Fig. 17-6G

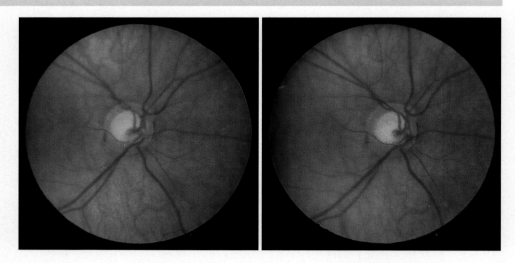

Right optic nerve head with cup-to-disc ratio of approximately 0.6 to 0.7. Glaucomatous optic nerve damage may increase the cup-to-disc ratio, as was the case in this patient with a history of glaucoma.

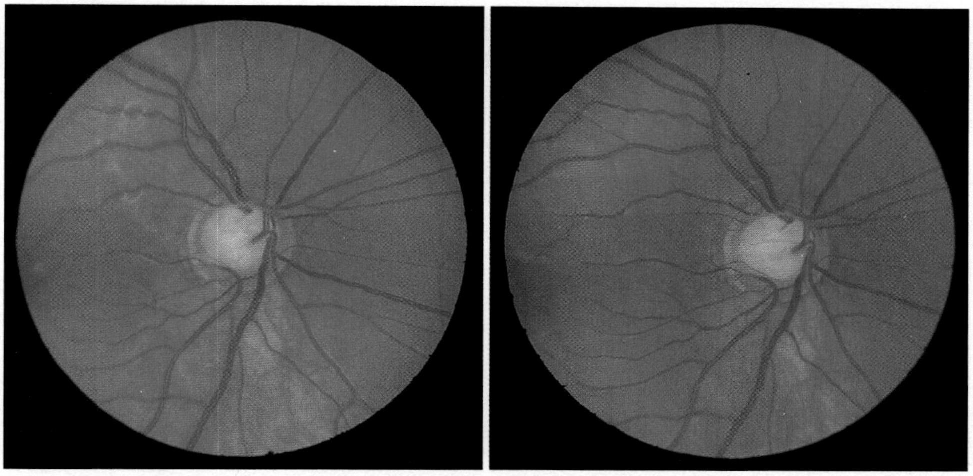

Fig. 17-6H

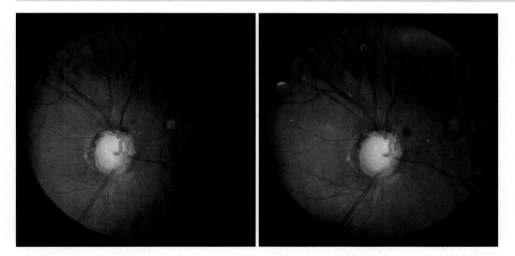

Right optic nerve head with cup-to-disc ratio of approximately 0.7 in a patient with a history of glaucoma.

Fig. 17-6I

Right optic nerve head with cup-to-disc ratio of approximately 0.8. This patient had a history of glaucoma.

Fig. 17-7

Optic disc drawings may be used to document the appearance of the optic nerve head.

Fig. 17-7A

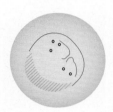

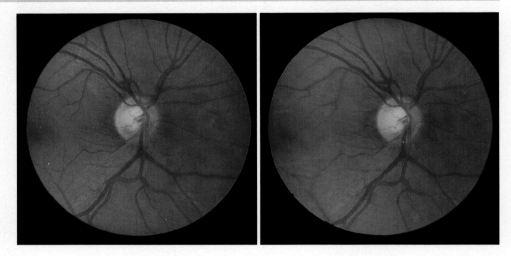

Right optic nerve head with a moderate-sized cup. Hatched lines in the drawing (left) indicate a sloping inferotemporal neural rim. Laminar pores are indicated by dots.

Fig. 17-7B

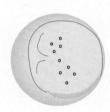

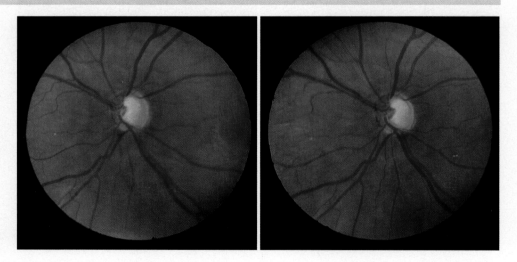

A large cup with a thin temporal neural rim in a glaucoma patient. Thinning of the neural rim extends nearly to the margins of the disc. Laminar pores are indicated by dots in the disc drawing (left).

Fig. 17-8

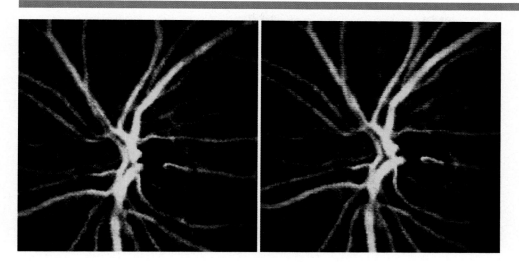

Computer-assisted enhancement of blood vessels. This figure shows a digitized stereoscopic image of a normal optic nerve with colors reversed and blood vessels enhanced. Several quantitative techniques have been described to assist in the analysis of the topography or appearance of the optic nerve head. (Images provided by Sherry L. Olson and Eric J. Donaldson, Mitre Corporation, Bedford, Massachusetts.)

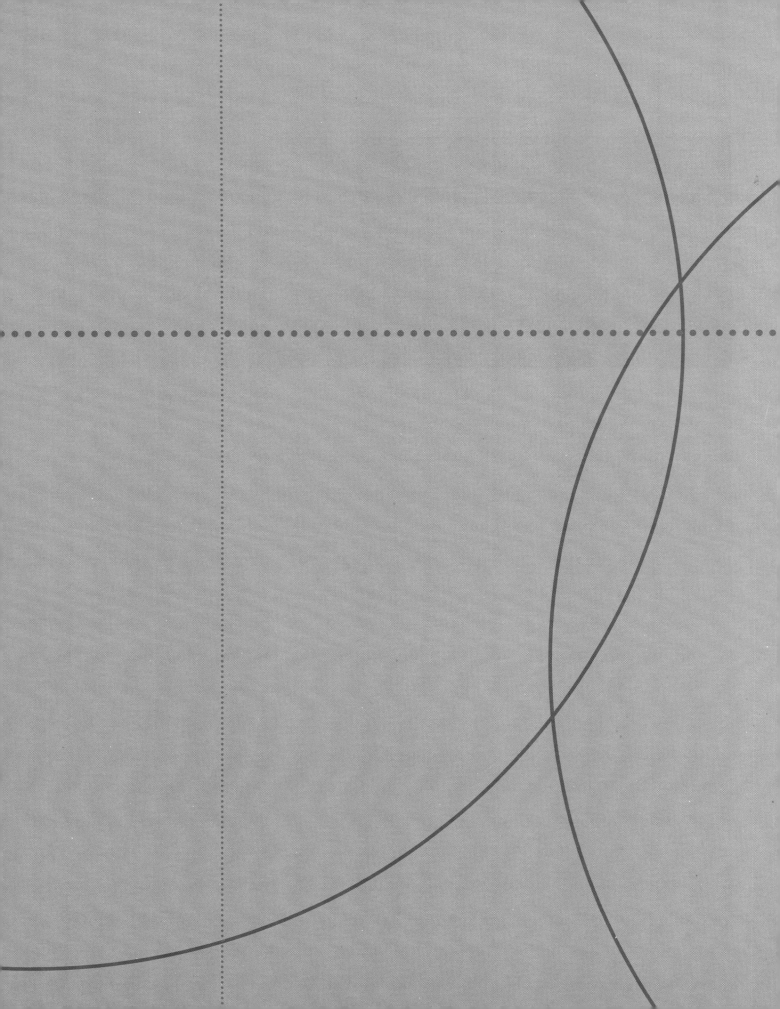

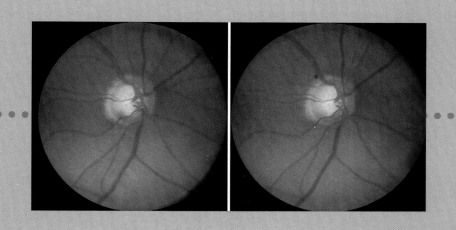

CHAPTER 18

GLAUCOMATOUS OPTIC NERVE

Ocular Hypertension

Ocular hypertension is a term that indicates elevated intraocular pressure, normal-appearing discs and visual fields, open angles, and no known ocular or systemic condition accounting for the increased pressure.[1] Elevated intraocular pressure is defined as greater than 21 mmHg, which is two standard deviations above the mean in population-based studies.[2] The prevalence of ocular hypertension is higher than predicted by this definition because the intraocular pressure in populations does not fit a gaussian distribution but instead is skewed toward the higher side.[2] Although only approximately 0.5% to 1% of ocular hypertensive patients per year develop visual field loss as detected by kinetic perimetry,[1] these patients may lose as many as 50% of their optic nerve axons despite having normal kinetic visual fields.[3] There is an increased risk for development of glaucoma in ocular hypertensive patients; however, in many of these patients, glaucomatous optic nerve damage does not develop. On initial clinical presentation, the normal-appearing optic nerve cannot distinguish patients who do not have glaucoma from those in whom glaucoma is developing or those in whom early subtle damage of the optic nerve has developed (Figs. 18-1 and 18-2). Currently, only continued clinical monitoring can identify patients without glaucoma and those with early glaucoma in whom glaucomatous changes of the optic nerve develop over time.

Glaucomatous Optic Nerve Cupping

Primary open-angle glaucoma is the most common form of glaucoma in the United States, accounting for 60% to 70% of the cases of glaucoma in this country.[1] This entity is a chronic, progressive optic neuropathy characterized by cupping and atrophy of the optic disc, visual field loss, open angles, elevated intraocular pressure, and no known contributing ocular or systemic conditions. Less commonly, progressive optic nerve cupping, visual field defects, open angles, and no other contributing ocular or systemic factors may occur in the absence of elevated intraocular pressure, which is an entity known as low-tension or normal-tension glaucoma.[4,5] Other glaucomas have been classified as "secondary" because physicians have at least partial understanding of underlying ocular or systemic causes of the glaucoma. Examples of secondary glaucomas include pigmentary glaucoma and pseudo-exfoliation glaucoma. Population studies have shown differences in the appearance of the optic nerve head in patients with different types of glaucoma.[6] However, there generally are no diagnostic findings in the optic nerve head that can clearly identify the type of glaucoma in any given individual.

At the time of clinical presentation of glaucoma patients, the appearance of the optic nerve head varies. There is no uniform pattern of glaucomatous cupping of the optic nerve head (Fig. 18-3). An abnormal optic nerve contour inevitably is found in all patients with glaucoma, and some of these patients can be placed in certain categories based on the appearance of their optic nerve head.[7,8] Focal tissue loss often may occur at the superior or inferior pole and with a relatively intact neural rim in other areas of the disc. Generalized enlargement of the optic cup may occur without a localized defect of the neural rim. Myopic glaucomatous discs may have large cups with myopic temporal crescents and additional evidence of glaucomatous damage. Also, senile sclerotic discs have been described, with saucerized and shallow cups, a "moth-eaten" appearance, a pale neural rim, and peripapillary chorioretinal atrophy.[9]

Identification of progressive changes of the contour of the optic nerve head permits diagnosis and appropriate management of glaucoma (Figs. 18-4 through 18-8). As emphasized by Spaeth, no single path to glaucomatous optic nerve damage occurs, but instead there are varying patterns by which the nerve becomes damaged.[10] At least four patterns of glaucomatous damage to the optic nerve have been identified by Spaeth, including (1) concentric enlargement of the cup, (2) focal extension of the cup or notching, (3) development of an acquired pit, and (4) development of pallor. One type of focal extension of the cup is vertical extension, which may occur early in the course of glaucomatous optic nerve damage (Fig. 18-9). An uncommon early pathologic change in the disc is a slight backward bowing in the periphery of a portion of the disc or of the whole disc, which has been termed "saucerization."[11] The contour of such a disc resembles the contour of a saucer (Fig. 18-10), in contrast with a marked excavation or undermining of the neural rim that more closely resembles the contour of a teacup.

Optic nerve cupping that results from chronic elevation of intraocular pressure and loss of nerve tissue is unlikely to reverse. In contrast, acute elevation followed by control of intraocular pressure may cause reversal of disc cupping.[12] The younger the patient, the more likely that the cupping will reverse after reduction of the intraocular pressure. Less dramatic reversal of cupping is expected in older patients presumably because of reduced elasticity of scleral tissue and the lamina cribrosa, which limits the normalization of the optic nerve head contour after surgical or medical lowering of the intraocular pressure.

Visual field defects due to glaucomatous optic nerve atrophy generally correspond to visible changes of the optic nerve head.[11] Glaucomatous optic nerve cupping in the inferotemporal region of the disc may produce a superior nasal step, a superior Bjerrum scotoma, or both (Fig. 18-11 through 18-15). Conversely, superotemporal excavation of the neural rim may result in an inferior Bjerrum scotoma, an inferior nasal step, or both (Fig. 18-16). The visual field defect associated with acquired optic nerve pits generally is a dense arcuate defect that extends close to fixation.[13] In eyes with extensive cupping and atrophy of the neural rim or in highly myopic eyes, the location and type of visual field defects often are difficult to predict based on the appearance of the optic nerve head (Fig. 18-17). Visual field changes that do not correspond with the appearance of the optic nerve head raise the possibility of nonglaucomatous abnormalities, including vascular occlusions, previous chorioretinitis, optic nerve drusen, brain tumors, and retinoschisis or other retinal abnormalities (Fig. 18-18).

Disc Hemorrhage

Disc hemorrhages were characterized by Drance[14] as typically linear, splinter- or flame-shaped hemorrhages located in the prelaminar area of the optic disc (Fig. 18-19). They often are located in the superficial nerve fiber layer, but may occur deeper in the nerve tissue. These hemorrhages may occur at any location around the disc rim, although they most commonly are located at the inferotemporal disc margin. Disc hemorrhages are transient and occur more frequently in eyes with low-tension glaucoma or primary-open angle glaucoma compared with ocular hypertensive and normal eyes.[14,15] They are uncommon in healthy eyes and may be associated with disease processes other than glaucoma, including posterior vitreous detachment, diabetic retinopathy, optic nerve drusen, papilledema, vasculitis, anticoagulation therapy, ischemic optic neuropathy, and retinal vein occlusion. In glaucomatous eyes, optic disc hemorrhages often are associated with progressive changes of the visual fields and optic nerve appearance.[16] Although there may be a delay after disc hemorrhage before progressive optic nerve or visual field changes are observed,[16] disc hemorrhage may be an important clinical finding when deciding whether to advance therapy in patients with glaucoma.

Abnormalities of Disc Vessels Associated with Glaucoma

The appearance of the vessels around the optic nerve head provides important information about optic disc contour.[17] Also, changes of the positions of vessels over time may indicate underlying glaucomatous atrophy of the optic nerve head. With progressive excavation and cupping of the optic nerve head, vessels in the region of the neural rim may bend noticeably. Progressive enlargement of the optic nerve cup causes the vessels to shift nasally, termed "nasalization" of vessels (Fig. 18-20). Vessels that pass circumferentially along the margin of the cup may become exposed in the depths of the cup as the neural rim recedes, which has been described as "baring of the circumlinear vessels" (Fig. 18-21). "Overpass" of vessels may occur with loss of neural rim tissue previously underlying the vessel, leaving the vessel appearing as suspended without any support (Fig. 18-22). If the neural rim is undermined, the part of the vessel in the area of the neural rim may be bent sharply in this crevice, which may give the vessels a "bayonet" appearance (Fig. 18-23). The caliber of retinal vessels may become narrowed in chronic glaucoma. Although the most common cause of optociliary vein is central retinal vein occlusion,[18] vascular shunts and collaterals may occur in glaucomatous optic nerve heads, presumably due to chronic venous stasis (Fig. 18-24). In neovascular glaucoma, neovascularization of the disc may be observed (Fig. 18-25).

Parapapillary Chorioretinal Atrophy

In some optic nerve heads, there is chorioretinal atrophy in the region bordering the disc (Fig. 18-26). This parapapillary chorioretinal atrophy has been classified into two zones: alpha and beta.[19] The peripheral zone (alpha) is an area of irregular hypopigmentation and hyperpigmentation with thinning of the chorioretinal tissue layer. Zone alpha may be directly in contact with the peripapillary scleral ring, or there may be another zone (beta) interposed between zone alpha and the edge of the disc. Zone beta is characterized by visible sclera and choroidal vessels, with an absence of pigmentation. When both zones are present, zone beta is adjacent to the edge of the disc, whereas zone alpha has a more peripheral position. The ophthalmoscopic appearance of zone beta is caused by complete loss of retinal pigment epithelium and choriocapillaris, whereas zone alpha is caused by irregularities of the retinal pigment epithelium.[20] Zones alpha and beta are considered distinct from the scleral crescent in eyes with high myopia and from the scleral crescent in eyes with tilted optic discs.

Zone alpha occurs up to five times more frequently compared with zone beta,[19] and both zones most frequently are positioned in the temporal horizontal sector.[21] In eyes with glaucomatous optic nerve atrophy, both zones are significantly larger, and zone beta occurs more often than in normal eyes.[21] These zones may occur adjacent to areas of excavation or thinning of the neural rim.[22-24] Progressive atrophy of the parapapillary retinal pigment epithelium may accompany glaucomatous optic nerve cupping[25] (Figs. 18-27 and 18-28). It is not clear whether preexisting parapapillary chorioretinal atrophy may predispose the eye to glaucomatous damage or whether this atrophy is part of the process of glaucomatous damage.

REFERENCES

1. Hoskins HD and Kass M: Becker-Shaffer's diagnosis and therapy of the glaucomas, ed 6, Philadelphia, Mosby, 1989, pp 277–307.

2. Wilson MR and Martone JF: Epidemiology of chronic open-angle glaucoma. In Ritch R, Shields MB, and Krupin T, editors: The glaucomas, ed 2, Philadelphia, Mosby, 1996, pp 753–768.

3. Quigley HA et al: Optic nerve damage in human glaucoma: II, the site of injury and susceptibility to damage. Arch Ophthalmol 99:635, 1981.

4. Werner EB: Normal-tension glaucoma. In Ritch R, Shields MB, and Krupin T, editors: The glaucomas, ed 2, Philadelphia, Mosby, 1996, pp 753–768.

5. Grosskreutz C and Netland PA: Low-tension glaucoma. Int Ophthalmol Clin 34:173, 1994.

6. Caprioli J: Correlation between optic disc appearance and type of glaucoma. In Varma R and Spaeth GL, editors: The optic nerve in glaucoma, Philadelphia, JB Lippincott Company, 1993, pp 91–98.

7. Spaeth GL: A new classification of glaucoma including focal glaucoma. Surv Ophthalmol 38:S9, 1994.

8. Nicolela MT and Drance SM: Various glaucomatous optic nerve appearances: clinical correlations. Ophthalmology 103:640, 1996.

9. Geijssen HC and Greve EL: The spectrum of primary open angle glaucoma: I, senile sclerotic glaucoma versus high tension glaucoma. Ophthalmic Surg 18:207, 1987.

10. Spaeth GL: Development of glaucomatous changes of the optic nerve. In Varma R and Spaeth GL, editors: The optic nerve in glaucoma, Philadelphia: JB Lippincott Company, 1993, pp 63–81.

11. Epstein DL: Chandler and Grant's glaucoma, ed 3, Philadelphia, Lea & Febiger, 1986, pp 14–101.

12. Hetherington J: Glaucomatous optic disc changes in infants. In Varma R and Spaeth GL, editors: The optic nerve in glaucoma, Philadelphia: JB Lippincott Company, 1993, pp 83–90.

13. Cashwell LF and Ford JG: Central visual field changes associated with acquired pits of the optic nerve. Ophthalmology 102:1270, 1995.

14. Drance SM: Disc hemorrhages in the glaucomas. Surv Ophthalmol 33:331, 1989.

15. Kitazawa Y, Shirato S, and Yamamoto T: Optic disc hemorrhage in low-tension glaucoma. Ophthalmology 93: 853, 1986.

16. Siegner SW and Netland PA: Optic disc hemorrhages and progression of glaucoma. Ophthalmology 103: 1014, 1996.

17. Airaksinen PJ, Tuulonen A, and Werner EB: Clinical evaluation of the optic disc and retinal nerve fiber layer. In Ritch R, Shields MB, and Krupin T, editors: The glaucomas, ed 2, Philadelphia, Mosby, 1996, pp 617–657.

18. Masuyama Y et al: Clinical studies on the occurrence and the pathogenesis of optociliary veins. J Clin Neuro-Ophth 10:1, 1990.

19. Jonas JB and Naumann GOH: The optic nerve: its embryology, histology, and morphology. In Varma R and Spaeth GL, editors: The optic nerve in glaucoma, Philadelphia: JB Lippincott Company, 1993, pp 3–26.

20. Kubota T, Jonas JB, and Naumann GO: Direct clinico-histological correlation of the parapapillary chorioretinal atrophy. Br J Ophthalmol 77:103, 1993.

21. Jonas JB et al: Parapapillary chorioretinal atrophy in normal and glaucoma eyes. Invest Ophthalmol Vis Sci 30:908, 1989.

22. Anderson DR: Correlation of the peripapillary anatomy with the disc damage and field abnormalities in glaucoma. Doc Ophthalmol Proc Ser 35:1, 1982.

23. Heijl A and Samander C: Peripapillary atrophy and glaucomatous visual field defects. Doc Ophthalmol Proc Ser 42:403, 1984.

24. Jonas JB and Naumann GOH: Parapapillary chorioretinal atrophy in normal and glaucoma eyes: II, correlations. Invest Ophthalmol Vis Sci 30:919, 1989.

25. Rockwood EJ and Anderson DR: Acquired peripapillary changes and progression in glaucoma. Graefes Arch Clin Exp Ophthalmol 226:510, 1988.

Optic nerve appearance of patients with ocular hypertension. These patients had normal vision fields, open angles by gonioscopy, and intraocular pressure greater than 21 mmHg. These images show normal-appearing optic nerves in these patients, although the size of the cup varies. The appearance of the optic nerve in these patients cannot distinguish those who are healthy from those with early glaucoma.

Fig. 18-1

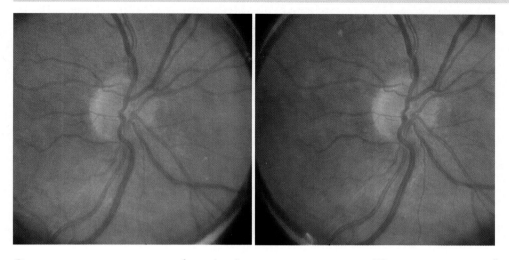

Fig. 18-1A

Optic nerve appearance of ocular hypertensive patient. The appearance of the optic nerve in Figs. 18-1A through 18-1D cannot distinguish those who are healthy from those with early glaucoma.

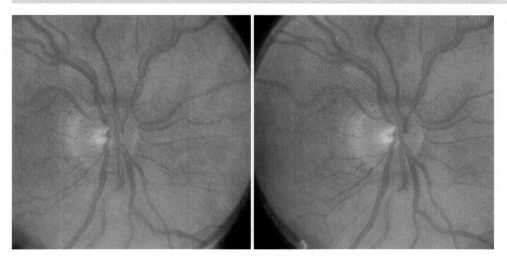

Fig. 18-1B

Optic nerve appearance of ocular hypertensive patient. The cup is slightly larger in this optic disc compared with the disc shown in Fig. 18-1A.

Fig. 18-1C

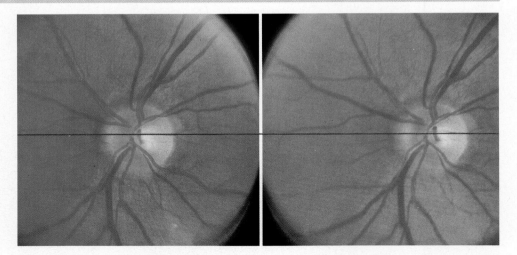

Optic nerve appearance of ocular hypertensive patient. The appearance of the optic disc cannot distinguish whether this patient has or does not have early glaucoma.

Fig. 18-1D

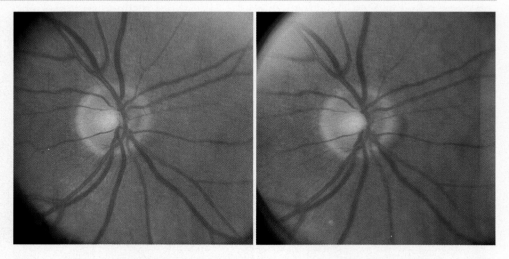

Optic nerve appearance of ocular hypertensive patient. Although the cup is larger than the cup shown in Figs. 18-1A through 18-1C, there are no findings in the optic disc that are pathognomonic for glaucoma.

Optic disc asymmetry in two eyes of the same patient.   **Fig. 18-2**

Fig. 18-2A

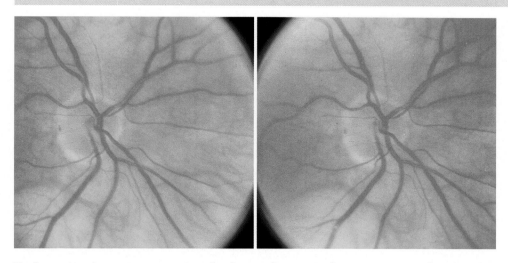

Right optic disc in a patient with elevated intraocular pressure and asymmetric appearance of the optic nerves. The angles were open by gonioscopy and the visual fields were normal.

Fig. 18-2B

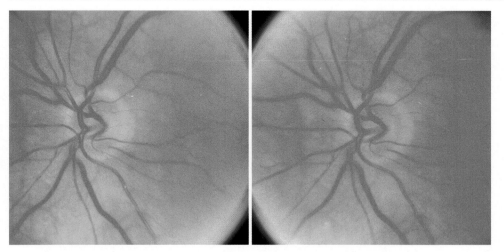

Left optic disc in the same patient shown in Fig. 18-2A. The left optic disc has an enlarged cup and nasalization of vessels. Although the asymmetric appearance is not common, the finding of disc asymmetry alone is not diagnostic of glaucoma. Subsequent examinations during a 10-year follow-up period, however, identified glaucomatous changes of the optic nerve head contour that were more pronounced in the left eye.

Fig. 18-3

Examples of the varied appearance of the optic nerve head in patients with glaucoma. Although the appearance and degree of neural rim loss may vary, there are no diagnostic findings of the optic nerve head that can identify the specific type of glaucoma in any given patient.

Fig. 18-3A

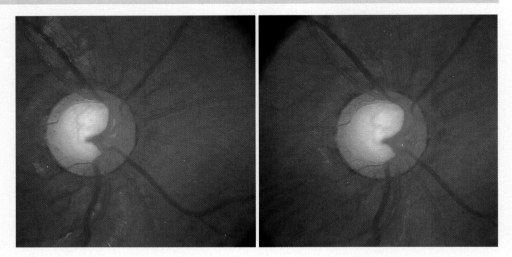

Generalized and concentric enlargement of the optic cup of the right eye. The neuroretinal rim is intact, the optic cup is deep, and there is no peripapillary atrophy.

Fig. 18-3B

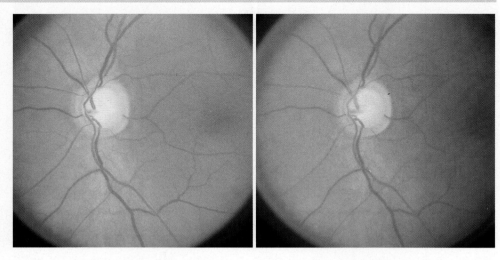

Generalized enlargement of the optic cup of the left eye with a thin but intact neuroretinal rim. The pores of the lamina cribrosa are visible at the base of the deep cup.

Fig. 18-3C

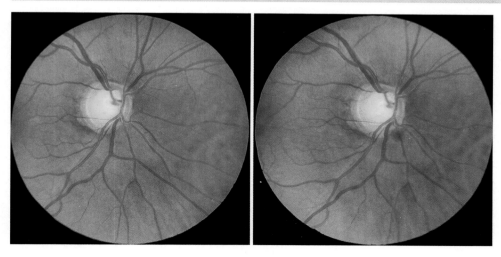

The right optic disc in a patient with primary open-angle glaucoma. The left optic disc of this patient is pictured in Fig. 18-3D.

Fig. 18-3D

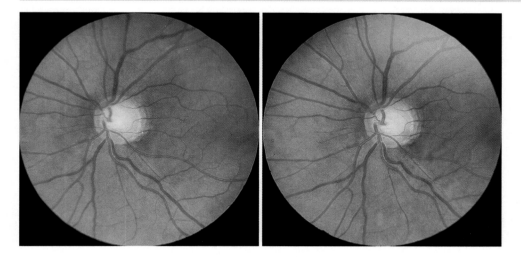

The left optic disc in a patient with primary open-angle glaucoma. The right optic disc of this patient is pictured in Fig. 18-3C. In this patient, there is enlargement of the optic cup in both eyes and peripapillary atrophy temporal to the disc, with a slightly larger cup (thinner neural rim) in the right eye compared with the left eye.

Fig. 18-3E

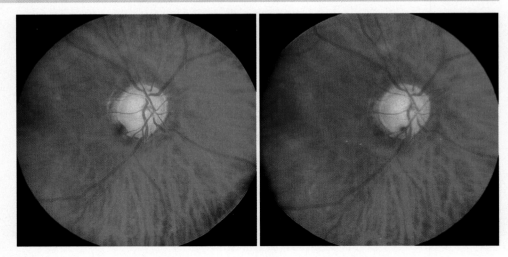

Right optic disc with a large cup and a thin neuroretinal rim, especially infero-temporally. The remaining optic nerve tissue is pale in appearance, and there is peripapillary atrophy temporal to the disc.

Fig. 18-3F

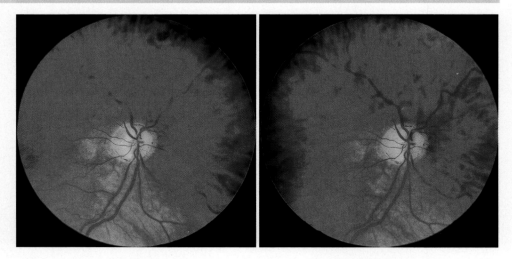

Right optic disc in a patient with low-tension glaucoma. The remaining neural tissue is pale (best visualized nasally) and thinned, especially inferiorly and slightly temporally. There is some shallow sloping nerve tissue remaining temporally, which has a moth-eaten appearance. Peripapillary atrophy can be seen around the disc. The superotemporal artery appears suspended over the disc without any underlying neural rim tissue ("overpass" of the vessel), and the caliber of this vessel is narrowed in areas. This so-called "senile sclerotic disc" may be found in patients with different types of glaucoma.

Fig. 18-3G

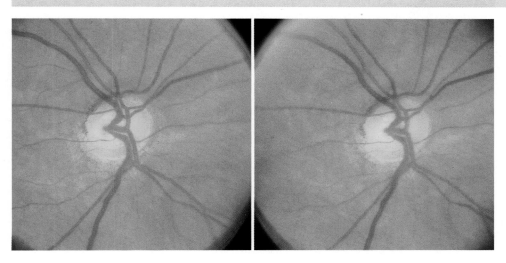

Right optic disc in a patient with primary open-angle glaucoma. The cup is enlarged and there is parapapillary atrophy. The remaining neural rim tissue is pale. The pores of the lamina cribrosa are visible through the nerve tissue at the inferior pole of the disc because of the pallor of the remaining neural rim tissue.

Fig. 18-3H

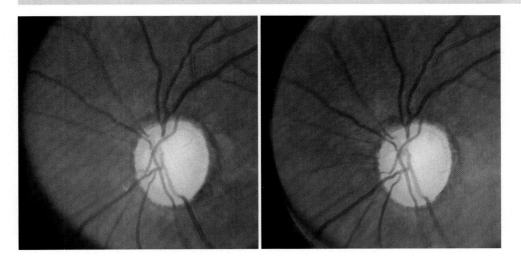

Left optic disc in a patient with primary open-angle glaucoma. There is advanced glaucomatous cupping with marked attenuation of the neuroretinal rim temporally.

Fig. 18-3I

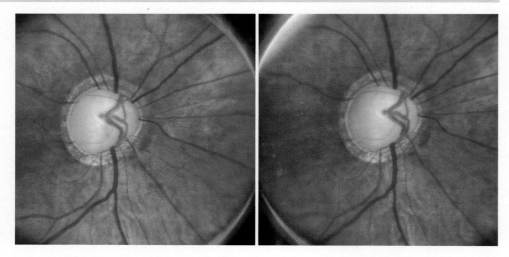

End-stage cupping in a patient with low-tension glaucoma. There is peripapillary atrophy and baring of circumlinear vessels at the superior and inferior poles of the disc.

Fig. 18-3J

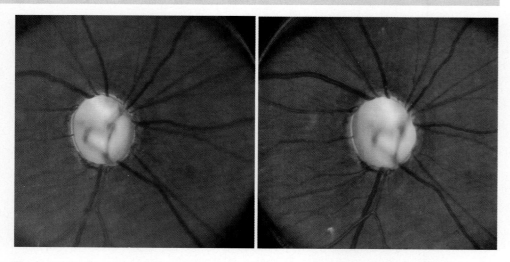

End-stage glaucomatous cupping in the right eye of a patient with primary open-angle glaucoma. The cup is excavated deeply and there is little remaining neural rim. Nerve fiber layer defects can be seen radiating from the optic disc.

Fig. 18-3K

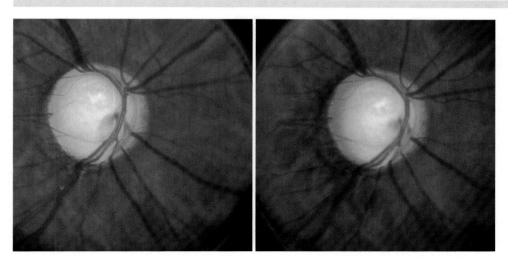

Right optic disc in a patient with juvenile open-angle glaucoma. The left optic disc of this patient is pictured in Fig. 18-3L. The optic cup is excavated deeply and peripapillary atrophy is present in both eyes. The right optic disc has a pale and severely attenuated neural rim, which can be visualized nasally and superiorly, but appears thin-to-absent inferotemporally.

Fig. 18-3L

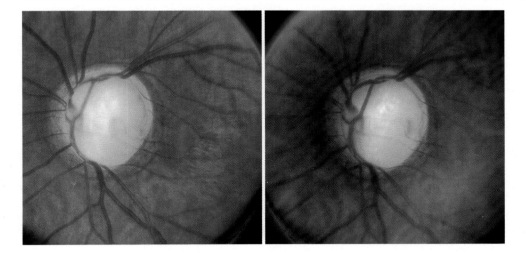

Left optic disc in patient with juvenile open-angle glaucoma. The right optic disc of this patient is pictured in Fig. 18-3K. The optic cup is excavated deeply and peripapillary atrophy is present in both eyes. The left optic disc has end-stage cupping with very little remaining neuroretinal rim.

Fig. 18-4   Progressive changes over time of the left optic disc in a patient with primary open-angle glaucoma.

Fig. 18-4A

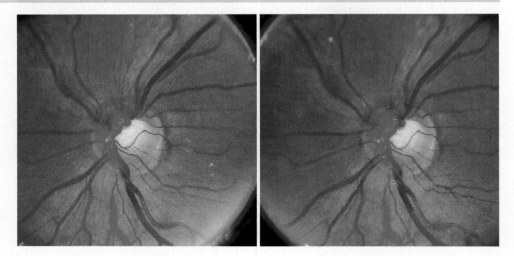

The initial photograph shows a deep cup, a sloped inferotemporal neural rim, and an area of peripapillary atrophy inferotemporally.

Fig. 18-4B

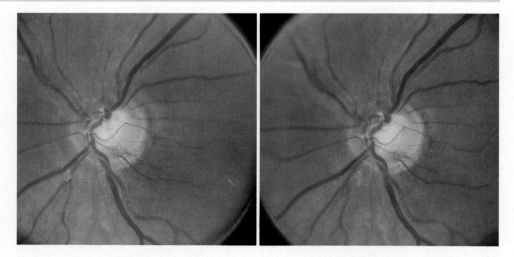

Comparison of Fig. 18-4A to this image obtained 12 years later shows several changes. The cup has become larger during the follow-up interval because of reduced thickness of the neural rim (note the change superonasally). The large-caliber vessels have been deflected nasally, and several vessels have changed position around the neuroretinal rim. There also is development of an acquired optic pit in the inferotemporal area, which can be identified by changes in the contour of the optic nerve tissue and the bending of the vessels in this region. The peripapillary atrophy in the inferotemporal area has increased in size, and there is a resolving disc hemorrhage inferotemporally in the more recent photograph.

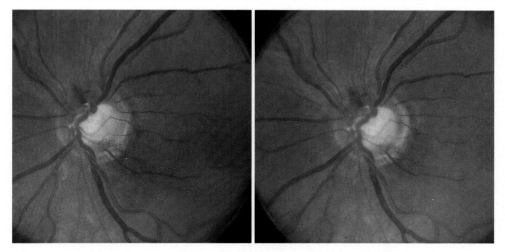

Fig. 18-4C

During the interval between Figs. 18-4A and 18-4B, multiple disc hemorrhages were observed in the inferotemporal region of the disc. Disc hemorrhages have been associated with progressive changes of the optic disc in patients with glaucoma.

Fig. 18-4D

Also during the interval between Figs. 18-4A and 18-4B, a disc hemorrhage was identified in the superonasal neuroretinal rim area. Disc hemorrhages are less common on the nasal side compared with the temporal side of the disc in patients with glaucoma.

Fig. 18-5   Progressive changes of the right optic disc in a patient with chronic open-angle glaucoma.

Fig. 18-5A

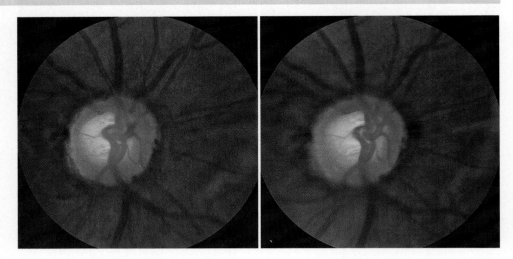

The initial photograph shows a large, deep cup with a symmetrical neural rim and minimal peripapillary atrophy.

Fig. 18-5B

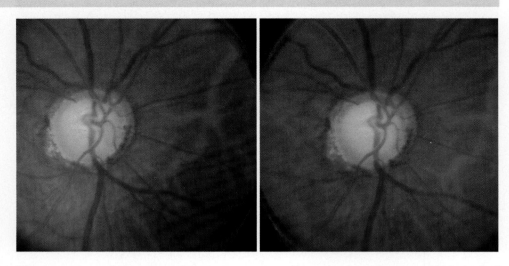

Thirteen years later, there is a concentric enlargement of the cup (thinning of the neural rim), a nasal shift of the disc vessels, and an increased area of peripapillary atrophy.

Progressive changes of the right optic disc in a patient with primary open-angle glaucoma.

Fig. 18-6

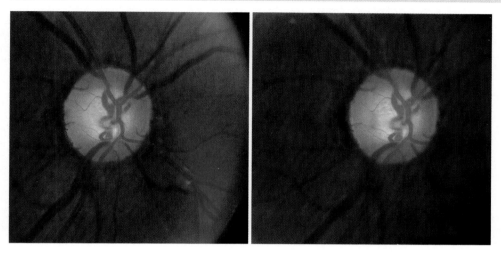

Fig. 18-6A

The initial photograph of the right optic disc in a patient with primary open-angle glaucoma.

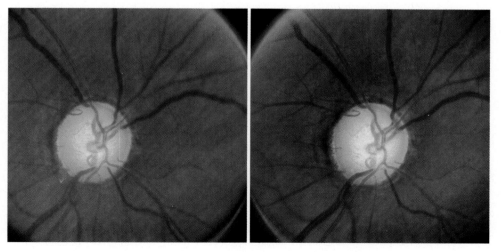

Fig. 18-6B

The patient after a 12-year interval. During this interval, there has been concentric enlargement of the cup. An area of focal thinning of the neural rim can be observed near a cilioretinal vessel in the superotemporal region. The bent portion of this vessel could not be visualized well before the loss of the overlying neural rim tissue.

Fig. 18-7

Changes over time of the left optic disc in a patient with elevated intraocular pressure.

Fig. 18-7A

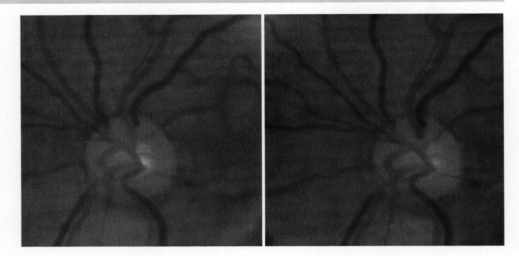

The initial photograph shows the appearance of the optic disc in a patient with elevated intraocular pressure and an otherwise normal ocular examination.

Fig. 18-7B

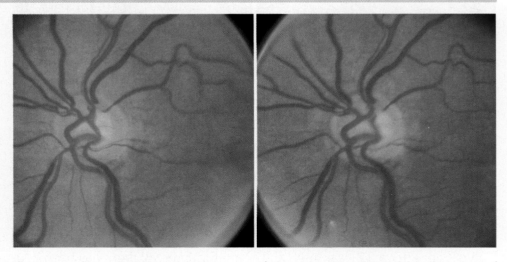

Five years later, there is enlargement of the optic cup. Note the thinning of the neural rim inferiorly and the changes of vessel positions.

Progressive changes with time in the right optic disc in a patient with low-tension glaucoma.

Fig. 18-8

Fig. 18-8A

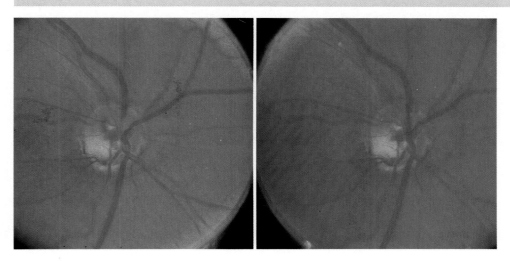

The initial photograph shows extension of the cup (notching) inferotemporally.

Fig. 18-8B

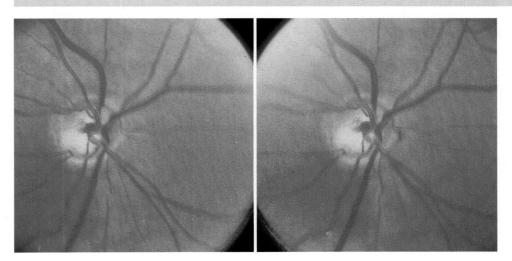

Seven years later, note thinning of the neural rim and shifts of the positions of blood vessels.

Fig. 18-8C

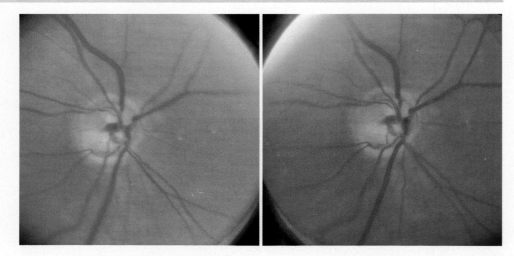

Fifteen years after the initial photograph, there is marked thinning of the neural rim and formation of an acquired optic pit inferotemporally. There was a dense superior arcuate visual field defect extending close to fixation. Despite numerous measurements during this period, the highest recorded intraocular pressure was 18mmHg.

Vertical extension of the optic cup.   **Fig. 18-9**

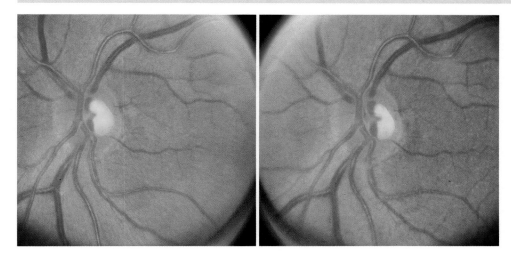

                    Fig. 18-9A

Left optic disc with an oval and vertically oriented cup in a patient with low-tension glaucoma. Focal extension of the cup inferiorly was noted on serial clinical examinations. The fellow eye had a thin inferotemporal neural rim and a glaucomatous visual field defect.

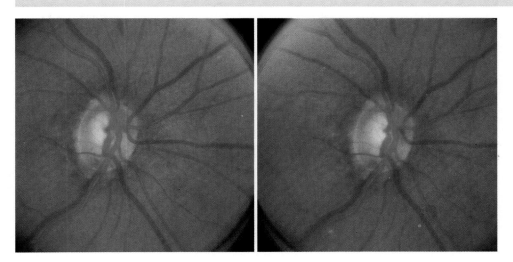

                    Fig. 18-9B

Right optic disc with a vertically oriented cup in a patient with primary open-angle glaucoma. The neural rim is thinnest at the superior pole, and there is a disc hemorrhage inferiorly.

Fig. 18-10   Saucerized optic discs.

Fig. 18-10A

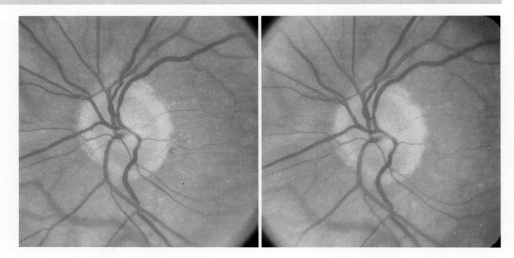

The neural rim is sloped toward the center of the left optic disc, more so on the temporal side of the disc. There is peripapillary atrophy around the margin of the disc and drusen visible in the retina surrounding the disc.

Fig. 18-10B

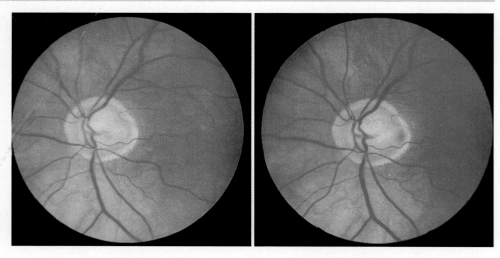

More pronounced posterior bowing of the left optic disc. Note that the pale neural rim is sloped rather than excavated sharply. Elschnig's ring and peripapillary atrophy can be viewed around the disc.

Optic nerve cupping associated with visual field defect.   **Fig. 18-11**

Fig. 18-11A

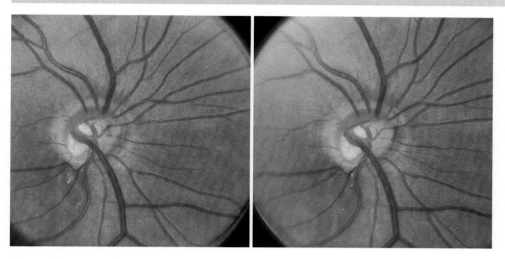

The right optic disc in a patient with low-tension glaucoma shows focal thinning of the neural rim inferotemporally.

Fig. 18-11B

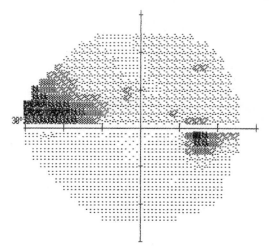

Automated perimetry shows a superior nasal step visual field defect.

Fig. 18-12   Glaucomatous optic nerve cupping associated with visual field defect.

Fig. 18-12A

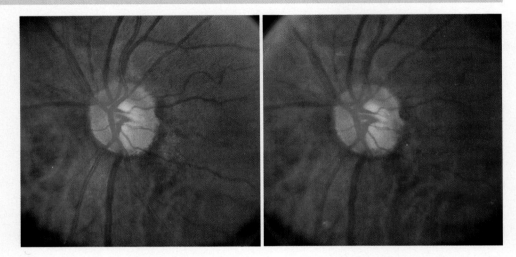

The left optic disc shows focal extension of the cup (notching) inferotemporally. Despite the marked tissue loss at the inferior pole, other areas of the
disc appear relatively undamaged.

Fig. 18-12B

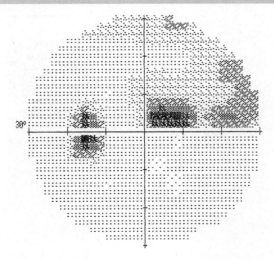

Automated perimetry shows a dense superonasal visual field defect extending
close to fixation.

Optic nerve cupping and visual field defect in a patient with combined mechanism glaucoma.

Fig. 18-13

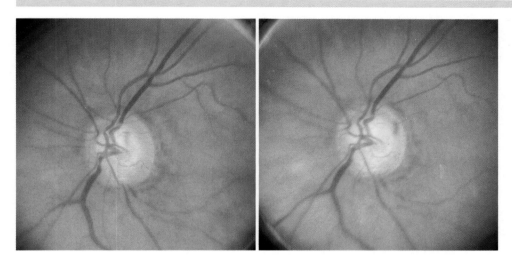

Fig. 18-13A

The neural rim is thinned at the inferior pole of the left optic disc. Note the bayonet vessel at the inferior pole of the disc, in the area of the thinned neural rim.

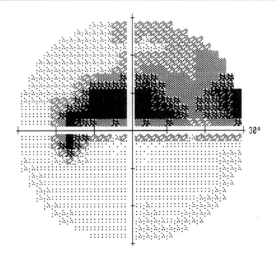
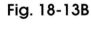

Fig. 18-13B

Automated perimetry shows a superior arcuate visual field defect.

Fig. 18-14   Cupping of the left optic disc and visual field defect in a patient with low-tension glaucoma.

Fig. 18-14A

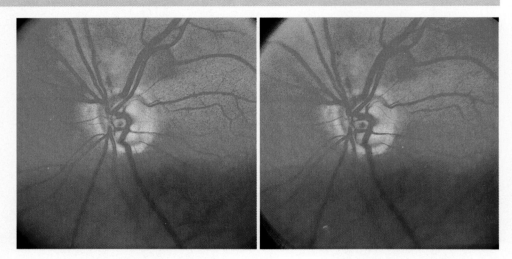

The neural rim is thinned and excavated at the inferior pole of the disc and thinned at the superior pole. There also is a disc hemorrhage in the superonasal quadrant of the disc.

Fig. 18-14B

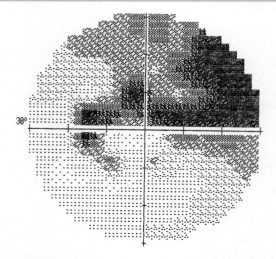

Automated perimetry shows a superior arcuate scotoma contiguous with a dense nasal scotoma. There also are inferior arcuate and nasal step defects that are less dense than those in the superior hemifield, giving the appearance of an asymmetric double Bjerrum (superior and inferior arcuate) scotoma.

Glaucomatous cupping of the right optic disc associated with visual field defect.

Fig. 18-15

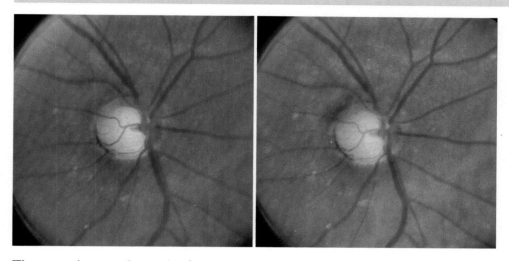

Fig. 18-15A

The neural rim is thinned inferiorly, whereas the superior neural rim is intact.

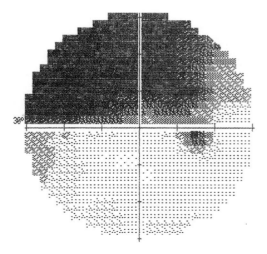

Fig. 18-15B

Automated perimetry shows a dense visual field defect in the superior hemifield.

Fig. 18-16   Visual field defect associated with glaucomatous cupping of the left optic disc in a patient with chronic open-angle glaucoma.

Fig. 18-16A

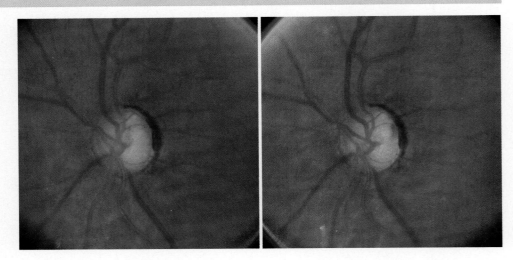

The neural rim is thinned and excavated superiorly and is thinned inferotemporally.

Fig. 18-16B

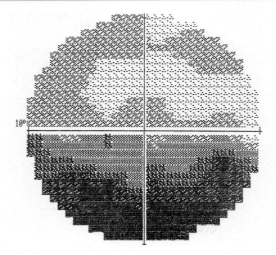

Automated perimetry shows a dense visual field defect in the inferior hemifield, with milder visual field changes in the superior hemifield.

Advanced glaucomatous optic nerve cupping and visual field loss in the right eye of a 9-year-old with steroid-induced glaucoma.

Fig. 18-17

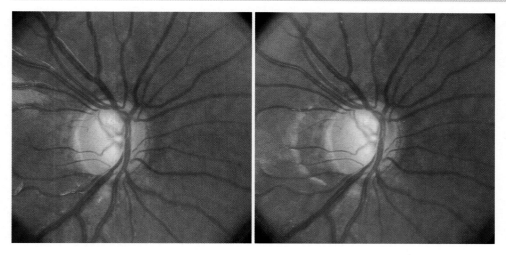

Fig. 18-17A

The right optic disc with a large cup with thinning of the neural rim at the superior and inferior poles of the disc.

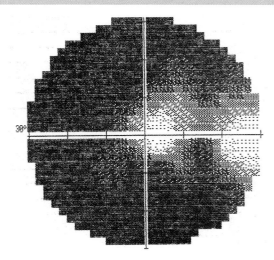

Fig. 18-17B

Automated perimetry shows advanced visual field loss superiorly and inferiorly extending to the blind spot. There are remaining central and temporal islands of vision.

Fig. 18-18   Visual field changes not corresponding to the appearance of the optic disc.

Fig. 18-18A

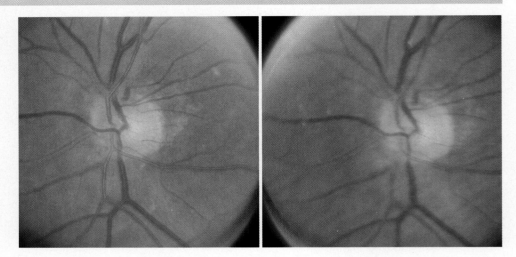

The left optic disc in a patient with a history of elevated intraocular pressure and a cerebrovascular accident. There is a disc hemorrhage at the superior pole of the disc, but the neural rim appears intact.

Fig. 18-18B

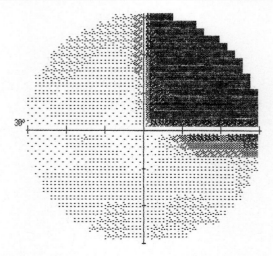

Automated perimetry of the left eye shows a dense superior nasal visual field defect.

Fig. 18-18C

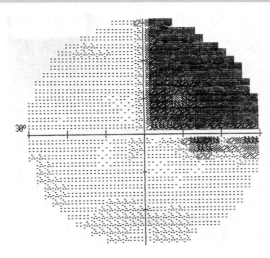

Automated perimetry of the right eye demonstrates the congruous right homonymous superior quadrantanopia due to a lesion in the left occipital lobe.

Disc hemorrhage in patients with glaucoma.   **Fig. 18-19**

Fig. 18-19A

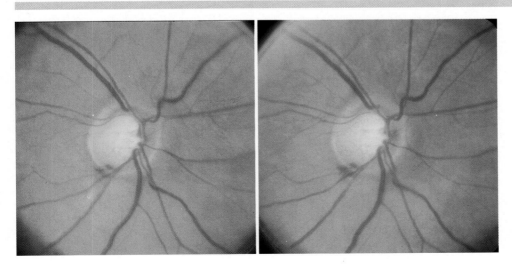

Inferotemporal disc hemorrhage of the right optic disc. This quadrant of the disc is the most common location of disc hemorrhages in glaucomatous eyes.

Fig. 18-19B

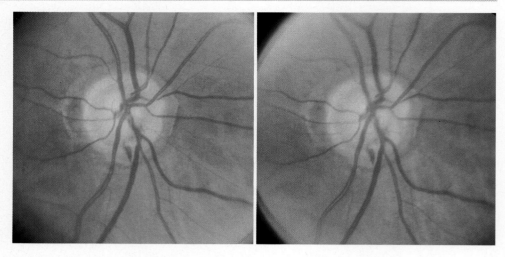

Disc hemorrhage at the inferior pole of the right optic disc.

Fig. 18-19C

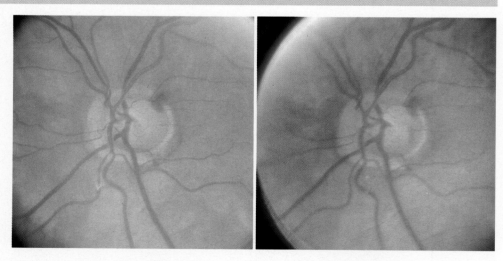

Superotemporal disc hemorrhage, left optic disc. There also is a resolving disc hemorrhage in the inferotemporal area.

Fig. 18-19D

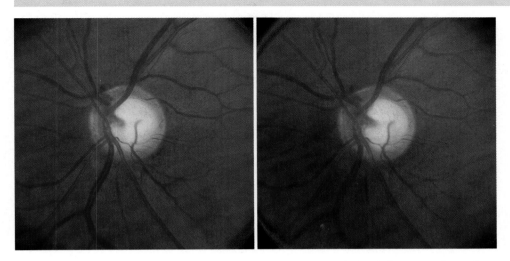

Disc hemorrhage located in the superonasal area of the left optic disc. Disc hemorrhages are less common on the nasal side compared with the temporal side of the disc in patients with glaucoma.

Fig. 18-19E

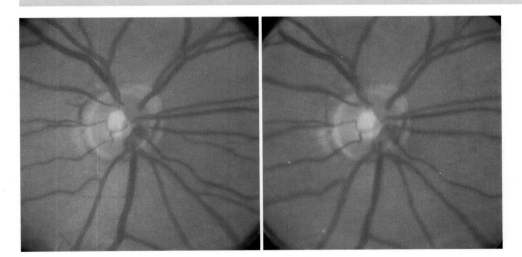

Disc hemorrhage in the inferonasal area of the right optic disc.

Fig. 18-19F

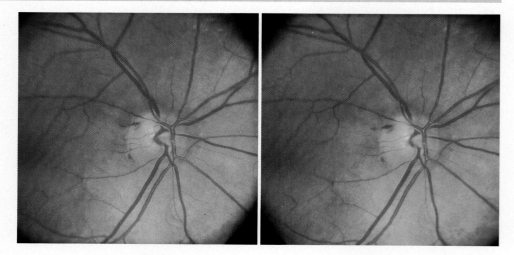

Disc hemorrhage located in the superotemporal quadrant of the right optic disc, adjacent to a focal extension of the cup (notch in the neural rim) at the superior pole of the disc. Disc hemorrhages often are associated with progressive changes of the visual field and optic disc contour.

Fig. 18-19G

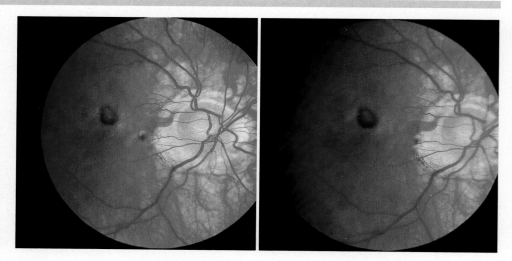

Right optic disc in a patient with myopia and primary open-angle glaucoma, with a choroidal vessel at the temporal margin of the disc in an area of peripapillary atrophy. A small-caliber vessel extending from the optic disc to the retina is anterior to the choroidal vessel. In the stereophotograph, this choroidal vessel can be distinguished readily from a disc hemorrhage.

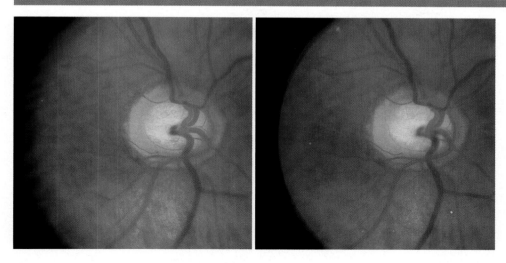

Right optic disc with nasalization of vessels. The vessels in the central area of the large cup are bent toward the nasal side of the disc.

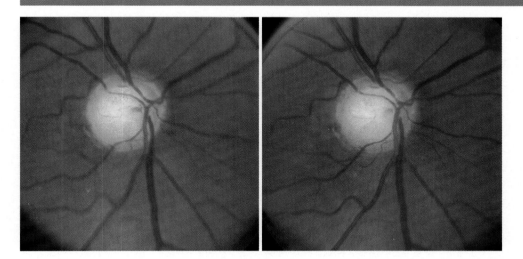

Right optic disc with baring of circumlinear vessel. The vessel passing circumferentially along the superior margin of the cup has become exposed in the depths of the cup, separate from the neuroretinal rim at the superior pole of the disc.

Fig. 18-20

Fig. 18-21

Fig. 18-22

"Overpass" of vessels in the optic disc.

Fig. 18-22A

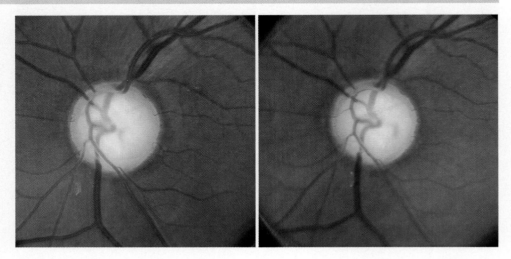

Left optic disc in a patient with advanced primary open-angle glaucoma with overpass of the artery at the inferior pole of the disc. The vessel appears suspended over the vein without any support.

Fig. 18-22B

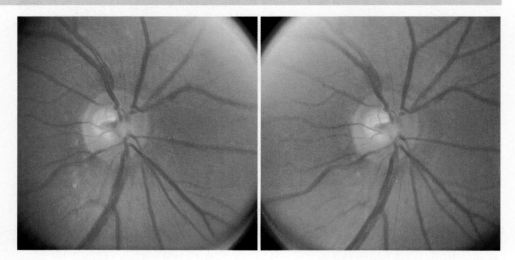

Right optic disc with overpass of small-caliber vessels extending toward the temporal pole of the disc. These vessels appear suspended in the cup without underlying support.

Fig. 18-23

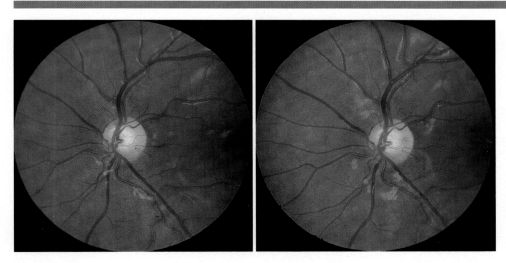

Left optic disc with a bayonet vessel bent sharply under the excavated neural rim at the superotemporal area of the disc. (Note also the superonasal excavation of the neural rim.) In some instances, the bent portion of the vessel may not be visible in the crevice behind the neural rim (see Fig. 18-13A). The shape of these vessels may resemble a bayonet mounted on a rifle.

Fig. 18-24   Formation of collateral vessels in the left optic disc of a patient with chronic open-angle glaucoma.

Fig. 18-24A

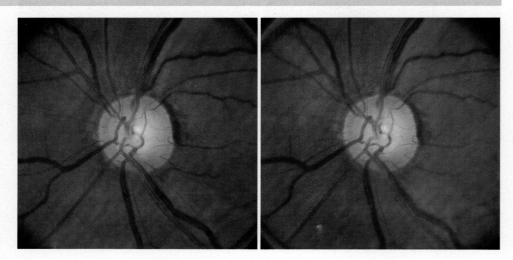

The initial stereophotograph of the disc.

Fig. 18-24B

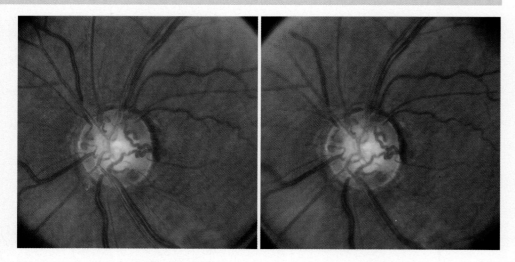

The appearance of the disc 10 years after the initial stereophotograph, with collateral veins evident. The patient was monitored approximately three times per year during the interval between photographs, and did not develop typical clinical findings associated with central retinal vein occlusion. There also has been mild progressive excavation of the neural rim during the interval between photographs.

Fig. 18-25

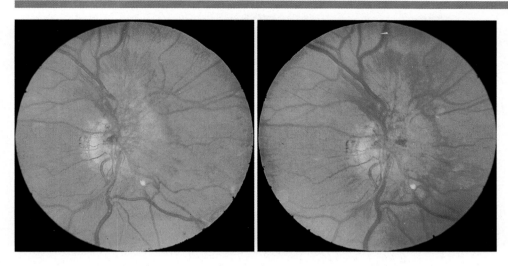

Neovascularization of the right optic disc in a diabetic patient with neovascular glaucoma.

Fig. 18-26   Parapapillary chorioretinal atrophy.

Fig. 18-26A

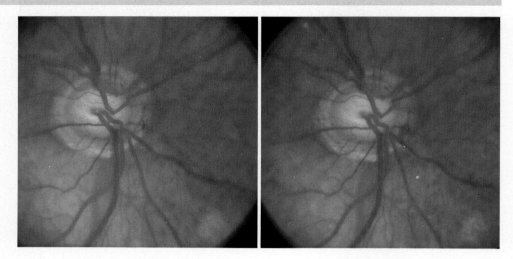

Right optic disc with parapapillary atrophy. The atrophy is predominately hypopigmentation with minimal irregular clumping of pigment.

Fig. 18-26B

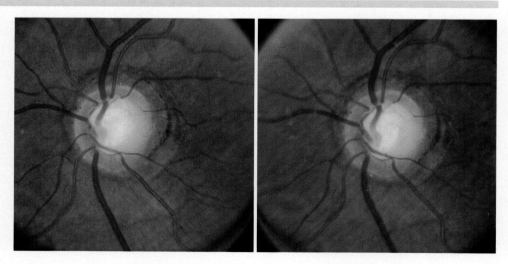

Left optic disc with parapapillary atrophy. There is irregular hypo- and hyper-pigmentation surrounding the disc (zone alpha), especially temporally and superiorly. (Note baring of circumlinear vessel deep in the cup inferiorly and a bayonet vessel at the inner margin of the neural rim superiorly and slightly temporally.)

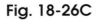

Fig. 18-26C

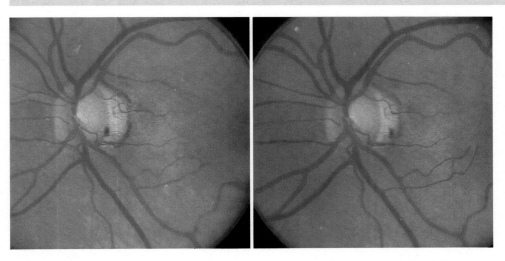

Left optic disc with parapapillary atrophy. The sclera and choroidal vessels are visible adjacent to the temporal margin of the disc (zone beta). Irregular pigmentation can be seen peripheral to the area of visible sclera and choroidal vessels.

Fig. 18-27   Progressive parapapillary chorioretinal atrophy in a patient with chronic open-angle glaucoma.

Fig. 18-27A

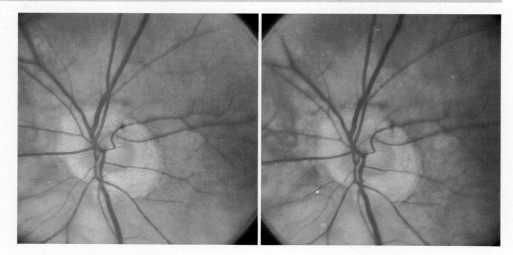

Initial photograph of left optic disc, with chorioretinal atrophy surrounding the disc. The sclera and choroidal vessels are visible adjacent to the disc margin (zone beta). Peripheral to zone beta, there is irregular hypopigmentation and hyperpigmentation (zone alpha).

Fig. 18-27B

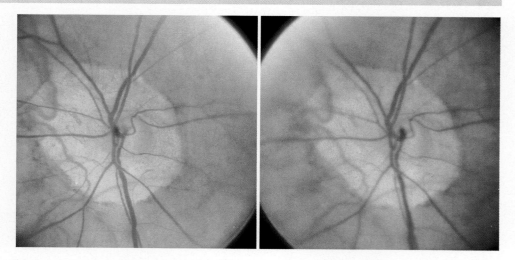

Eight years after the initial photograph, there is enlargement of the area of parapapillary atrophy. The neural rim also has thinned and the cup has enlarged during this interval (note changes of the position of vessels and the contour of the neural rim at the superior and inferior poles of the disc).

Progressive parapapillary atrophy in a patient with pigmentary glaucoma.   **Fig. 18-28**

Fig. 18-28A

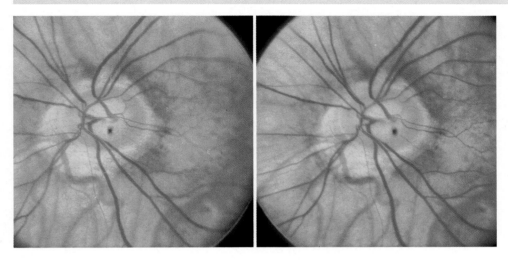

Initial photograph of the left optic disc, with chorioretinal atrophy around the disc, with the largest area of atrophy inferonasal to the disc.

Fig. 18-28B

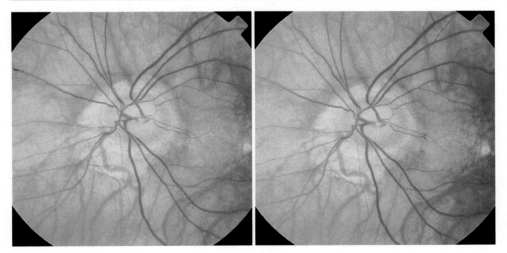

Five years after the initial photograph, there is enlargement of the area of parapapillary atrophy, especially in the area inferonasal to the disc. Note the position of the zone of atrophy relative to the vessels around the disc, particularly to the bend of the large choroidal vessel inferonasal to the disc.

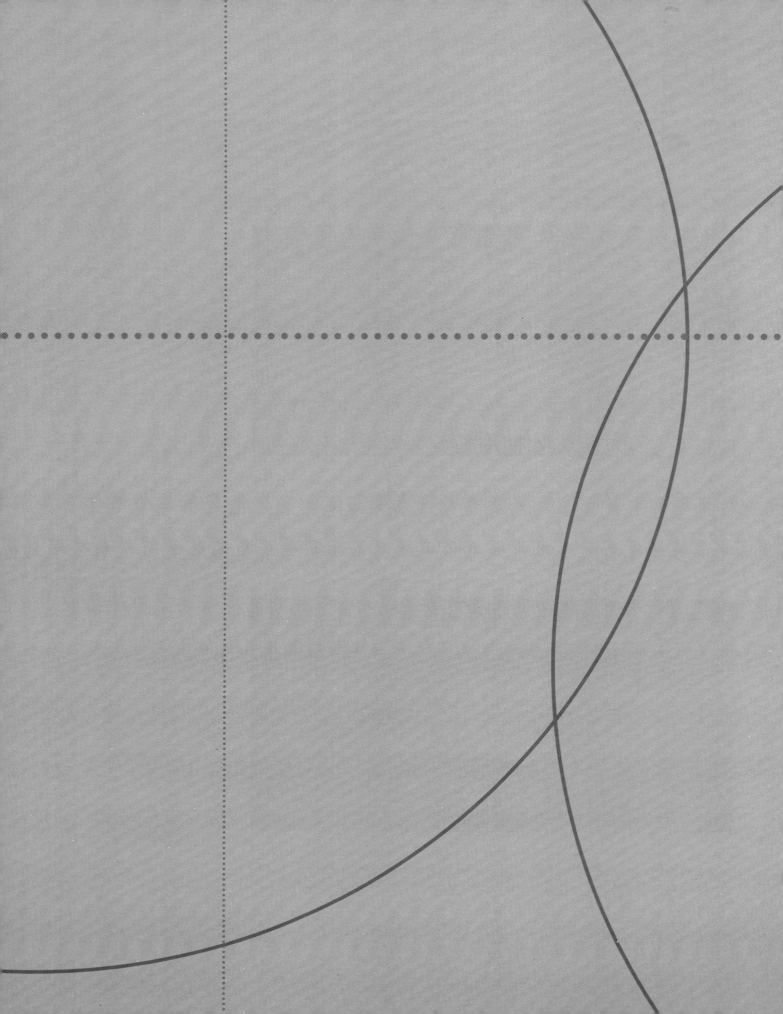

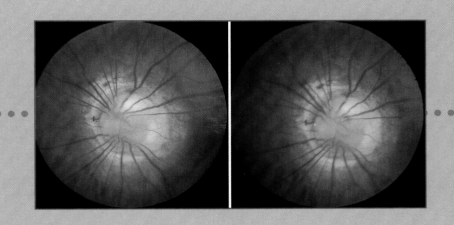

CHAPTER 19

PSEUDOGLAUCOMATOUS
OPTIC NERVE ABNORMALITIES

Congenital Anomalies

In adults, *congenital optic nerve pits* may be confused with acquired optic nerve pits, which may develop in glaucoma patients. Inferotemporal congenital pits, in particular, may be difficult to distinguish from glaucomatous change. Congenital optic pits are more likely than acquired pits to be localized, have gray or black color, and have adjacent peripapillary atrophy (Fig. 19-1). Fluorescein angiography of congenital optic pits often shows early hypofluorescence that progresses to late hyperfluorescence. Most importantly, congenital optic pits are present at birth and are nonprogressive, in contrast with the changes that occur over time in acquired pits. This change with time may be difficult or impossible to assess in adult patients, especially those presenting for an initial evaluation.

The incidence of congenital pits is approximately 1 in 11,000 patients.[1] These pits are located on the temporal aspect of the disc in the majority of cases and are positioned centrally in approximately one quarter.[2] The color is gray in approximately 60%, yellow or white in approximately 30%, and black in approximately 10%.[2] Unilateral involvement is observed in 85% of cases, and, excluding central optic pits, adjacent peripapillary retinal pigment epithelial changes are seen in the majority of patients. The visual field may be normal or abnormal and may not correlate with the size and location of the pit. Visual field defects associated with congenital optic pits include arcuate scotomas, peripheral defects or paracentral scotomas, generalized constriction, and nasal or temporal steps.

Patients with congenital pits of the optic nerve head may develop serous detachment of the macula (Fig. 19-2). Temporal location and larger pit size are predisposing factors for macular retinal detachment.[2] Spontaneous reattachment of the macula occurs in 25% or more of patients with optic pits.[3] With prolonged delay in reattachment, cystic degeneration and macular hole formation may occur. The origin of the fluid is unclear, but it appears to arise from either the cerebrospinal fluid or the vitreous. Prolonged retinal detachment may lead to vision loss in affected patients.

An *optic nerve coloboma* may occur alone or in combination with retinochoroidal or iris colobomata. Typical colobomata result from failure of the embryonic fissure to close along the inferonasal aspect of the optic cup and stalk. There is evidence suggesting that optic nerve pits, morning glory syndrome, and congenital tilted disc syndrome are all variants of the process that produces typical colobomata.[4] An isolated optic nerve coloboma is a rare congenital anomaly.

Characteristic ophthalmoscopic features of optic nerve colobomata include enlargement of the disc, partial or complete excavation usually inferiorly, blood vessels positioned at the borders of the defect, and a glistening white surface (Fig. 19-3). Peripapillary hypo- and hyperpigmentation commonly are present, and glial-appearing tissue may fill part of the defect. The abnormality may be unilateral or bilateral, both eyes probably are more commonly involved than one alone, and when bilateral, they often are asymmetric. The visual acuity in affected eyes is variable, ranging from normal to no light perception, although optic nerve coloboma usually is associated with some decrease in visual acuity.[5]

The visual field defects that occur in eyes with optic nerve coloboma can mimic those found in glaucomatous eyes (Fig. 19-4). When visual loss is severe, only an inferotemporal island of vision may remain.[5] Visual loss also may occur due to progressive loss of tissue from the colobomatous nerve. These eyes may be susceptible to glaucomatous-appearing damage, even at normal intraocular pressure.[6]

Other ocular and systemic abnormalities may occur in association with optic nerve colobomata. Secondary nonrhegmatogenous retinal detachments may develop, often in the second or third decades of life. These detachments can resolve spontaneously, although complete blindness results in approximately one quarter of cases.[5] In addition to retinal detachment, iris and retinochoroidal colobomas are associated with optic nerve coloboma (Fig. 19-5). Numerous systemic abnormalities have been reported in association with ocular colobomata, including dermatologic, gastrointestinal, genitourinary, central nervous system, musculoskeletal, and nasopharyngeal defects.[7]

The *morning glory syndrome* has several identifying features, including an enlarged and excavated disc, a central core or white or gray glial-appearing tissue, and a surrounding annulus of variably hypopigmented subretinal tissue (Fig. 19-6). The retinal vessels are positioned at the margins of the disc, often are sheathed, and have a straightened, radial appearance. This rare anomaly is named for its resemblance to the morning glory flower.

The morning glory anomaly usually is unilateral and often is associated with myopia.[5] Visual acuity may be decreased, particularly in unilateral cases, with amblyopia possibly playing a role in the visual loss. Like optic nerve pits, nonrhegmatogenous retinal detachments may occur in the posterior pole and can resolve spontaneously. Unlike optic nerve pits, these detachments may extend to involve most of the fundus. Although visual field defects may appear glaucomatous, the characteristic appearance of the disc usually identifies this anomaly.

The *tilted disc syndrome* occurs in approximately 1% to 2% of the population[8] and has a characteristic ophthalmoscopic appearance (Fig. 19-7). The long axis of the oval optic disc is obliquely directed, and the upper and temporal regions of the disc are anterior to the inferonasal area.[3] The retinal vessels may emerge from the disc tissue in the superotemporal area rather than nasally (situs inversus). There is an area of hypopigmentation and staphylomatous ectasia in the direction of the tilt, generally inferonasal to the optic disc. The majority of affected eyes have myopic astigmatism. The disc margin may be ill defined and elevated superiorly, which may be mistaken for papilledema. In contrast with the glaucomatous optic disc, the tilted disc usually is not excavated but is elevated superiorly and colobomatous inferiorly instead.[5] Central vision may be decreased mildly, and visual field defects, when present, tend to cross the vertical midline.

Optic nerve hypoplasia is characterized by small diameter of the optic nerve head, a low disc/artery ratio, and abnormal termination of the retinal pigment epithelium at the disc border, known as the "double ring sign" (Fig. 19-8). The yellow-gray peripapillary halo bridges the sclera-lamina cribrosa junction and the termination the retinal pigment epithelium.[3] Optic nerve hypoplasia may be associated with midline cerebral defects, such as lack of the septum pellucidum (DeMorsier's syndrome). Optic nerve hypoplasia may be unilateral or bilateral and is associated with significant reduction of vision in most affected eyes. The visual fields may be abnormal, but the clinical features of this syndrome readily distinguish it from glaucoma. Disc contour may be difficult to evaluate in eyes with optic nerve hypoplasia and elevated intraocular pressure.

Hereditary Optic Neuropathies

Hereditary optic neuropathies cause bilateral, symmetrical visual loss, although the loss of vision may not be simultaneous in both eyes. Loss of central vision is associated with dyschromatopsia and altered appearance of the optic nerve head. In the late stages of these neuropathies, there often is pallor of the optic nerve, which may be associated with excavation of the neural rim. Alterations of the visual field are common. Classification of the hereditary optic neuropathies is based on the genetics of transmission (whether mendelian or mitochondrial), the age of presentation, and the presence of associated neurologic or systemic abnormalities.[9]

Dominant optic atrophy, which is transmitted according to the mendelian rules, has been divided into two entities, depending on the age of onset. In the infantile variant, loss of visual acuity and color vision is severe, and nystagmus usually develops in affected patients. In the juvenile variant, loss of vision is mild to moderate, and blue-yellow dyschromatopsia develops in patients. Recessive optic atrophy presents with moderate loss of visual acuity (to the 20/200 level) and color vision, with nystagmus developing in approximately half of affected individuals.[9] A variant of recessive optic atrophy has been described by Behr, which is associated with ataxia, mental retardation, pyramidal tract dysfunction, increased tonicity, urinary incontinence, and pes cavus.[10] The clinical course usually is stable after the development of vision abnormalities.

Dominant and recessive optic atrophy are associated with pallor and excavation of the neural rim of the optic nerve head. Often, the pallor and excavation is sectoral and generally is temporally located. Visual field abnormalities commonly include central, centrocecal, or paracentral scotomas.[9] Depression of temporal isopters can occur, although peripheral fields generally are normal. The family history, normal intraocular pressure, early age of onset, and central vision loss generally distinguish these hereditary optic atrophies from glaucoma.

Recessive optic atrophy may develop in association with diabetes mellitus, known as Wolfram syndrome. This entity also is associated with development of diabetes insipidus and neurosensory hearing loss (Fig. 19-9), which is known by the commonly accepted acronym DIDMOAD (*diabetes insipidus, diabetes mellitus, optic atrophy,* and *deafness*). The loss of visual acuity and color vision often is severe, and the clinical course is progressive. Visual field changes include central scotomas and general constriction. The optic atrophy often is marked and may be accompanied by excavation of the neural rim.

Leber's optic neuropathy affects predominantly young adult males, causing acute or subacute loss of central vision at first usually in one eye, and later affecting both eyes. Its inheritance does not conform to mendelian laws, because the disease is transmitted by an abnormality of mitochondrial DNA. Vision loss and color vision loss often are severe, nystagmus is not expected, and the chronic clinical course is not progressive.[9] During the acute phase of the optic neuropathy, there is a swelling of the nerve fiber layer around the disc, with tortuous, telangiectatic vessels on and around the disc. In this pseudodisc edema, there is no leakage of dye on fluorescein angiography. In the late, atrophic phase, there is loss of previously telangiectatic vessels, pallor, and excavation of the neural rim (Fig. 19-10). Optic nerve head contour changes are common in Leber's hereditary optic neuropathy,[11] although the clinical characteristics of this entity generally are distinct from glaucoma.

Optic Nerve Drusen

Drusen may be visible as discrete crystalline structures in the optic nerve head, sometimes located deep within the optic nerve (Fig. 19-11). They may cause a swollen appearance of the optic nerve head and may be associated with anomalous tortuosity of the retinal vessels. These "hyaline bodies" are amorphous, partly calcified, extracellular deposits in the prelaminar portion of the optic nerve.[3] Because of their calcium content, optic disc drusen may be visualized with orbital computed tomography.[12] Drusen may be associated with visual field changes (Figs. 19-12 and 19-13), which may be especially difficult to interpret in the setting of simultaneous occurrence of drusen and elevated intraocular pressure.[13]

Drusen may cause slow progressive loss of visual fields or acute vision loss.[3] Chronic visual field loss characteristically is inferonasal in a nerve fiber layer distribution, and occasionally central visual loss may occur. Acute vision loss usually is caused by subretinal exudation and hemorrhage, often associated with peripapillary choroidal neovascularization. Occasionally, acute visual loss is associated with disc swelling, flame-shaped hemorrhages, and even cotton-wool spots, presumably due to disruption of the optic nerve blood supply. Drusen also may be associated with vision loss because of retinal vein or artery occlusion.

Toxic Optic Neuropathy, Methanol Toxicity

A variety of toxins and deficiencies can cause optic neuropathy (Fig. 19-14). Visual loss usually is painless, bilateral, and progressive, with central or cecocentral scotoma, and optic atrophy occurs in the late stage.[14] In intoxications, loss of vision may be rapid, and disc edema may be observed quickly after exposure to the toxin.

Methanol is a well-known optic nerve toxin. Poisoning occurs after accidental or intentional ingestion of as little as half an ounce of methanol. Accidental poisoning may occur after ingestion of contaminated home-distilled liquor. Toxic metabolites of methanol appear to inhibit cytochrome oxidase and other oxidative enzymes in the optic nerve, causing retrolaminar optic nerve swelling, axonal compression, and disc edema.[14] Symptoms develop within 18 to 48 hours after the ingestion of methyl alcohol, and fundoscopic examination shows edema and hyperemia of the optic disc and engorgement of the retinal veins. Patients with dilated, fixed pupils usually die or suffer severe visual damage. In milder cases, a dense cecocentral scotoma, nerve fiber bundle defects, and peripheral field constriction are frequent visual field defects. Optic atrophy develops in 1 to 2 months, and optic nerve cupping that is similar in appearance to glaucomatous optic nerve atrophy may develop.

Compressive Lesions

Compressive lesions of the optic nerve or chiasm may cause optic neuropathy (Fig. 19-15), which can resemble glaucomatous cupping.[15] Although glaucomatous optic atrophy usually can be distinguished from compressive lesions of the chiasm and optic nerve by clinical examination, some patients with nonglaucomatous excavation of the neural rim and normal intraocular pressure may be diagnosed mistakenly with low-tension glaucoma.[16,17] Evidence of compressive intracranial lesions or hydrocephalus was found in 2 of 53 patients referred for evaluation for low-tension glaucoma.[18] Similarly, 8 of 141 subjects (6%) suspected of having glaucoma by optic nerve screening subsequently were found to have intracranial lesions.[19]

In addition to changes of the contour of the optic nerve head, visual field defects that resemble those found in glaucomatous eyes can be caused by compressive lesions of the optic nerve.[20] Compressive lesions may be especially difficult to recognize clinically in patients with elevated intraocular pressure. A compressive lesion should be considered in patients with visual fields that do not correspond to the appearance of the optic nerve head and in patients suspected of having low-tension glaucoma. In patients with normal intraocular pressure and cupping of the optic nerve head, a computed tomography scan is indicated when the patient is younger than expected, when there is lack of correspondence of the appearance of the discs and the visual fields, and when there is significant asymmetry of the optic nerve heads, optic nerve head pallor, pain, or dyschromatopsia.

Ischemic Optic Neuropathy

Anterior ischemic optic neuropathy causes visual loss and optic disc swelling (Fig. 19-16). Two variants can occur: an idiopathic or a giant-cell arteritic type. The giant-cell arteritic variant generally occurs in a slightly older population than the idiopathic type, and the arteritic type is associated with elevation of the Westergren erythrocyte sedimentation rate. Visual loss can be mild, but in more than half of the cases, visual acuity is 20/200 or worse. Visual field abnormalities commonly include centrocecal scotomas and altitudinal defects.

Within several months after the onset of visual loss, the disc develops generalized or segmented pallor. Although disc pallor is the prominent finding, optic nerve cupping sometimes follows acute ischemic insults to the optic nerve (Fig. 19-17).[21–23] An interesting syndrome of acute optic nerve infarction followed by nonprogressive optic nerve cupping has been described.[24] Cupping of the optic nerve may be more common after the arteritic type of ischemic optic neuropathy compared with the idiopathic type.[25,26] A history of hypotensive episode (hemodynamic crisis) was found in some patients with glaucomatous-appearing optic nerve cupping.[27] However, prospective studies of patients with acute blood loss in shock have not provided supportive evidence linking hypotension to glaucomatous optic nerve atrophy.[28]

Other Causes of Optic Nerve Cupping

Certain types of glaucoma may not be diagnosed during the initial clinical evaluation of a patient with optic nerve cupping and normal intraocular pressure. The intraocular pressure may be elevated intermittently in some glaucomas, including intermittent angle-closure glaucoma, glaucomatocyclitic crisis, and glaucoma associated with uveitis. Some glaucomas may be difficult to diagnose when they are seemingly in remission. This may occur with corticosteroid-induced glaucoma and uveitis or trauma. Patients may have normal intraocular pressure and nonprogressive optic nerve damage associated with pigment dispersion syndrome.[29] In these patients, previous elevated intraocular pressure may have caused optic nerve damage. Primary open-angle glaucoma may be masked by diurnal intraocular pressure changes or by oral beta-adrenergic antagonist. Nonglaucomatous abnormalities other than those described in this chapter may be associated with optic nerve cupping, including inflammatory or infectious optic neuropathies and vascular abnormalities. Syphilis, anemia, and carotid obstruction are examples of abnormalities that have been associated with glaucomatous-appearing optic nerve atrophy.[18] A careful clinical history and examination usually can distinguish glaucomatous from nonglaucomatous causes of optic nerve cupping.

REFERENCES

1. Kranenburg EW: Crater-like holes in the optic disc and central serous retinopathy. Arch Ophthalmol 64:912, 1960.

2. Brown GC, Shields JA, and Goldberg RE: Congenital pits of the optic nerve head: II, clinical studies in humans. Ophthalmology 87:51, 1980.

3. Gass JDM: Stereoscopic atlas of macular diseases, ed 3, St. Louis: CV Mosby Company, 1987, pp 727–765.

4. Apple DJ: New aspects of colobomas and optic nerve anomalies. Int Ophthalmol Clin 24:109, 1984.

5. Brown GC: Differential diagnosis of the glaucomatous optic disc. In: Varma R and Spaeth GL: The optic nerve in glaucoma, Philadelphia: JB Lippincott Company, 1993, pp 99–112.

6. Savell J and Cook JR: Optic nerve colobomas of autosomal-dominant heredity: a report on three families. Arch Ophthalmol 94:395, 1976.

7. Robb RM: Developmental abnormalities of the eye affecting vision in the pediatric years. In: Albert DM and Jakobiec FA, editors: Principles and practices of ophthalmology, Philadelphia: WB Saunders Company, 1994, pp 2791–2798.

8. Riise D: The nasal fundus ectasia. Acta Ophthalmol Suppl 126:5, 1975.

9. Katz B: Hereditary optic neuropathies. In Albert DM and Jakobiec FA, editors: Principles and practice of ophthalmology, Philadelphia: WB Saunders Company, 1994, pp. 2593–2599.

10. Behr C: Die komplizierte, hereditär-familiäre optikusatrophie des kindesalters: ein bisher nicht beschriebener symptomkomplex. Klin Monatsbl Augenheilkunde 47:38.

11. Ortiz RG et al: Optic disc cupping and electrocardiographic abnormalities in an American pedigree with Leber's hereditary optic neuropathy. Am J Ophthalmol 113:561, 1992.

12. Ramirez H, Blatt ES, and Bibri NS: Computed tomographic identification of calcified optic nerve drusen. Radiology 148:137, 1983.

13. Samples JR et al: Optic nerve head drusen and glaucoma. Arch Ophthalmol 103:1678, 1985.

14. Lessell S: Toxic and deficiency optic neuropathies. In Albert DM and Jakobiec FA, editors: Principles and practice of ophthalmology, Philadelphia: WB Saunders Company, 1994, pp 2599–2604.

15. Bianchi-Marzoli S et al: Quantitative analysis of optic disc cupping in compressive optic neuropathy. Ophthalmology 102:436, 1995.

16. Trobe JD et al: Nonglaucomatous excavation of the optic disc. Arch Ophthalmol 98:1046, 1980.

17. Gittinger JW et al: Glaucomatous cupping: sine glaucoma. Surv Ophthalmol 25:383, 1981.

18. Stewart WC and Reid KK: Incidence of systemic and ocular disease that may mimic low-tension glaucoma. J Glaucoma 1:27, 1992.

19. Shiose Y et al: New system for mass screening of glaucoma, as part of automated multiphasic health testing services. Jpn J Ophthalmol 25:160, 1981.

20. Hupp SL et al: Nerve fiber bundle visual field defects and intracranial mass lesions. Can J Ophthalmol 21:231, 1986.

21. Levene RZ: Low-tension glaucoma: a critical review and new material. Surv Ophthalmol 24:621, 1980.

22. Drance SM: Disc hemorrhages in the glaucomas. Surv Ophthalmol 33:331, 1989.

23. Quigley HA and Anderson DR: Cupping of the optic disc in ischemic optic neuropathy. Trans Am Acad Ophthalmol Otolaryngol 83:755, 1977.

24. Lichter PR and Henderson JW: Optic nerve infarction. Trans Am Ophthalmol Soc 75:103, 1977.

25. Doro S and Lessell S: Cup-disc ratio and ischemic optic neuropathy. Arch Ophthalmol 103:1143, 1985.

26. Sebag J et al: Optic disc cupping in arteritic anterior ischemic optic neuropathy resembles glaucomatous cupping. Ophthalmology 93:357, 1986.

27. Drance SM: Some factors in the production of low tension glaucoma. Br J Ophthalmol 56:229, 1972.

28. Jampol LM, Board RJ, and Maumenee AE: Systemic hypotension and glaucomatous changes. Am J Ophthalmol 85:154, 1978.

29. Ritch R: Nonprogressive low-tension glaucoma with pigmentary dispersion. Am J Ophthalmol 94:190, 1982.

Fig. 19-1   Congenital optic nerve pits.

Fig. 19-1A

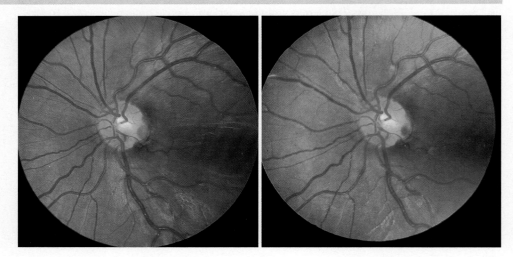

Congenital optic pit at the inferotemporal margin of the left optic disc. The pit is pale gray in color and is adjacent to an area of peripapillary hyper- and hypopigmentation.

Fig. 19-1B

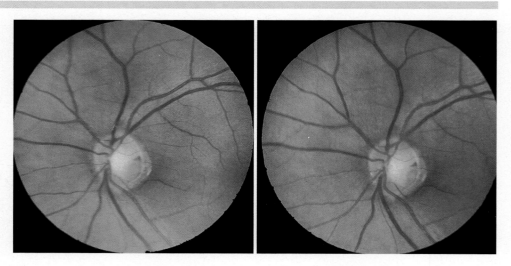

Gray-colored congenital optic pit at the inferotemporal margin of the left optic disc, which is adjacent to an area of peripapillary atrophy.

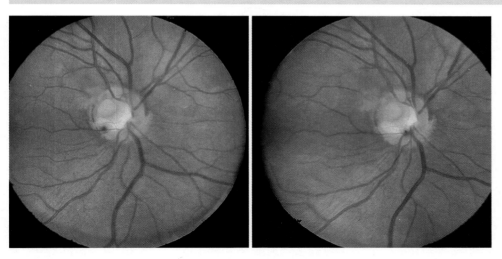

Fig. 19-1C

Congenital optic pit in the superotemporal area of the right optic disc. The neural rim is intact peripheral to the pit, and the peripapillary atrophy is not more pronounced adjacent to the pit than in other areas temporal to the disc. This optic pit is located slightly more centrally than the examples shown in Figs. 19-1A and 19-1B.

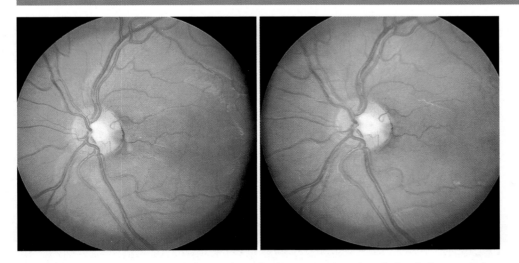

Fig. 19-2

Congenital optic nerve pit located at the temporal pole of the left optic disc associated with a serous detachment of the macula.

Fig. 19-3   Optic nerve coloboma.

Fig. 19-3A

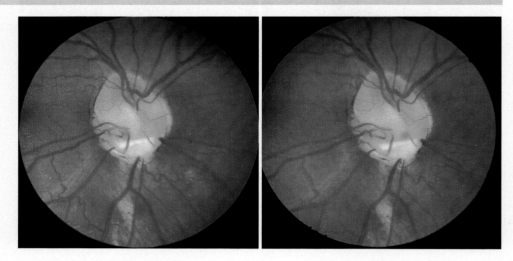

Optic nerve coloboma of the right optic disc, involving the inferior pole of the disc. Note the glistening white surface in the area of the coloboma.

Fig. 19-3B

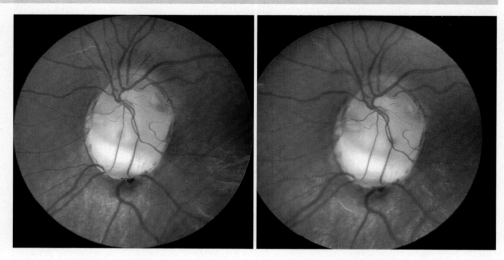

Optic nerve coloboma of the left optic disc. The disc is enlarged, the nerve is excavated inferiorly, and the inferior pole is white in color. There is increased peripapillary hyperpigmentation adjacent to the coloboma. Note the localized excavation inside the neural rim in the superotemporal area, which has the appearance of an optic pit.

Fig. 19-3C

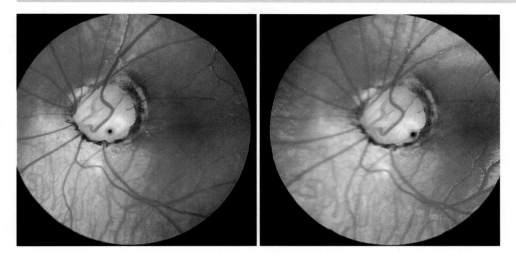

Optic nerve coloboma of the left disc. The entire disc is involved, with excavation of the disc and peripapillary hyper- and hypopigmentation.

Fig. 19-4

Visual field defect associated with left optic nerve coloboma.

Fig. 19-4A

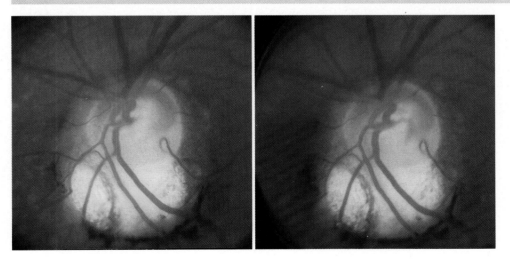

Enlarged optic disc with the coloboma involving the inferior pole of the disc. There also is peripapillary hyper- and hypopigmentation and an inferior retinochoroidal coloboma.

Fig. 19-4B

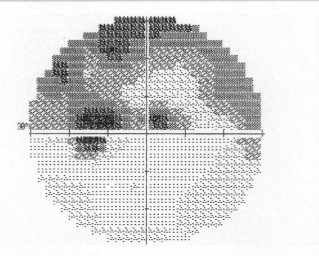

Automated perimetry of the left eye showing arcuate defect in the superior hemifield.

Fig. 19-5

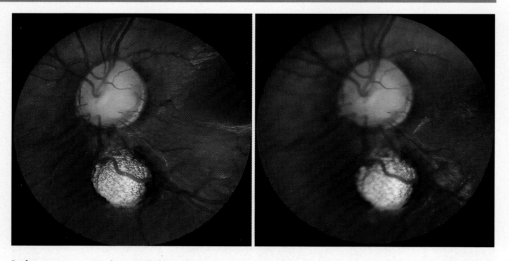

Inferior retinochoroidal coloboma associated with optic nerve coloboma involving the inferior pole of the left optic disc.

Morning glory anomaly.   **Fig. 19-6**

Fig. 19-6A

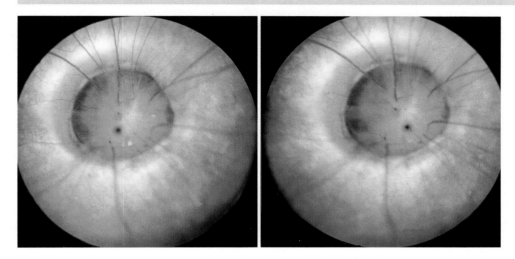

Morning glory anomaly with an enlarged disc, a central core of gray and white glial-appearing tissue, and a surrounding ring of variably pigmented subretinal tissue. The vessels are positioned toward the margin of the disc; some are sheathed and have a straightened, radial appearance.

Fig. 19-6B

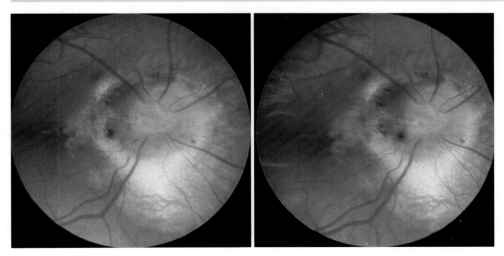

Morning glory anomaly of the right optic disc. The disc is enlarged and surrounded by a ring of variably pigmented subretinal tissue. The vessels are positioned toward the margin of the disc, some are sheathed, and they have a somewhat radial appearance. There is white glial-appearing tissue in the central area of the disc.

Fig. 19-7

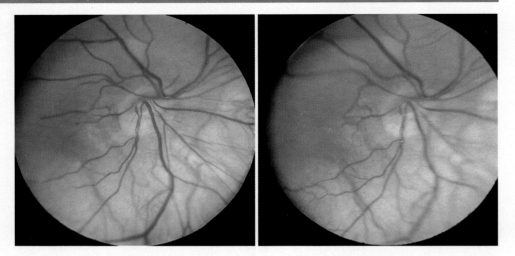

Tilted disc anomaly. The long axis of the right optic disc is obliquely directed, and the superotemporal pole is anterior to the inferonasal pole. There is
an area of hypopigmentation and ectasia inferonasal to the optic disc, in the
direction of the tilt.

Fig. 19-8

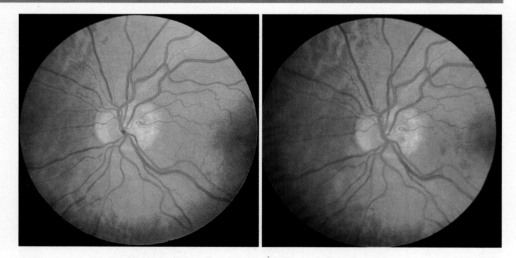

Optic nerve hypoplasia. The optic disc has a small diameter, a low disc/artery
ratio, and a yellow ring surrounding the disc (double ring sign). The peripapillary halo may be gray.

Recessive optic atrophy associated with diabetes mellitus. This patient had diabetes insipidus, diabetes mellitus, optic atrophy, and deafness (known as DIDMOAD).

Fig. 19-9

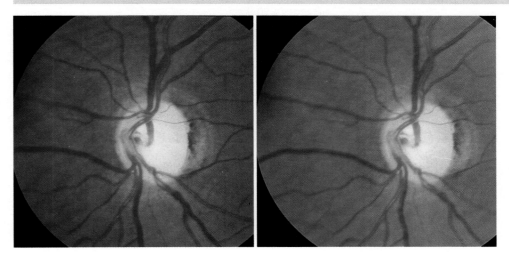

Fig. 19-9A

Left optic disc showing an enlarged cup, pale remaining neural rim, visible pores of the lamina cribosa, and peripapillary atrophy.

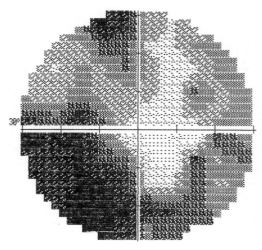

Fig. 19-9B

Automated perimetry shows extensive visual field loss.

Fig. 19-10

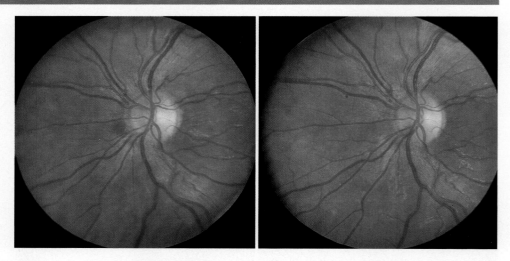

Leber's optic neuropathy. There is pallor and mild excavation of the temporal neural rim of the left optic disc.

Fig. 19-11   Optic nerve drusen.

Fig. 19-11A

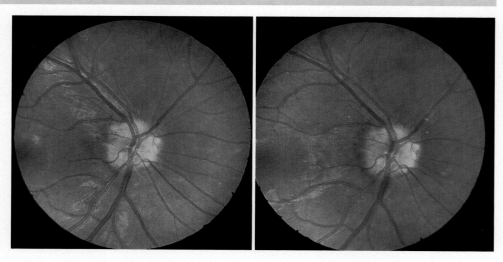

Right optic disc with drusen, which are most readily visible along the nasal margin of the optic disc.

Fig. 19-11B

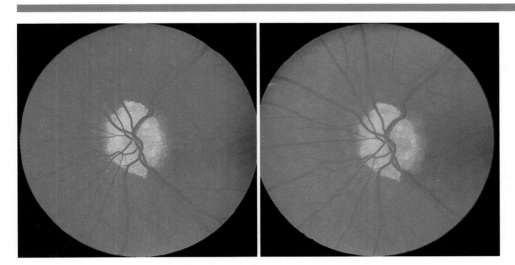

Crystalline-appearing drusen of the right optic disc.

Fig. 19-11C

Left optic disc containing a large number of drusen.

Fig. 19-12   Optic nerve drusen associated with visual field defect.

Fig. 19-12A

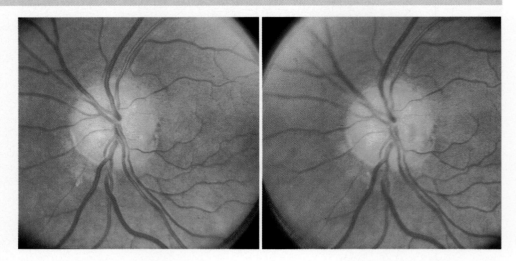

Left optic disc with white crystalline-appearing drusen embedded in the optic nerve tissue.

Fig. 19-12B

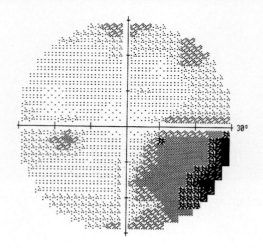

Automated perimetry showed an inferonasal visual field defect, which resembles a glaucomatous nasal step visual field defect.

Optic nerve drusen associated with visual field defect.

Fig. 19-13

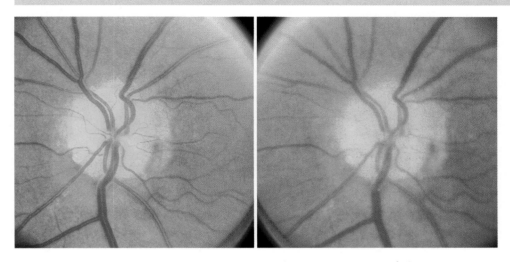

Fig. 19-13A

Left optic disc with drusen, causing a swollen appearance of the optic nerve head.

Fig. 19-13B

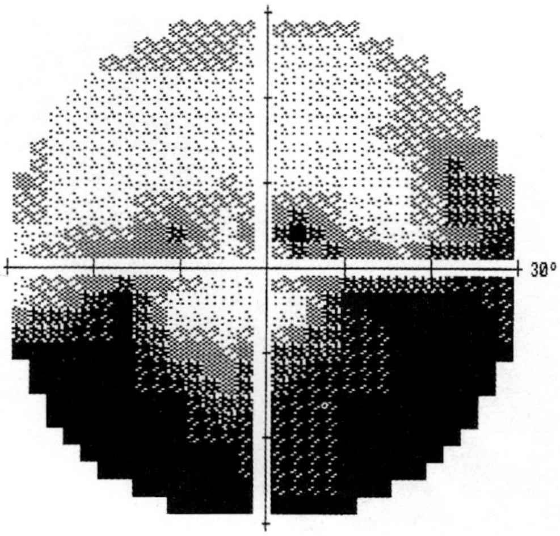

Automated perimetry shows glaucomatous-appearing dense inferior arcuate and less-dense superior arcuate (double Bjerrum) visual field defects contiguous with a superonasal visual field defect.

Fig. 19-14   Toxic optic neuropathy.

Fig. 19-14A

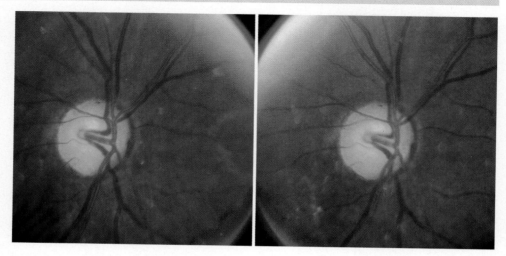

Right optic disc in a patient with a history of optic neuropathy due to ethambutol toxicity. In the acute stage, visual loss and dyschromatopsia developed.
In the chronic stage (shown), the neural rim is pale.

Fig. 19-14B

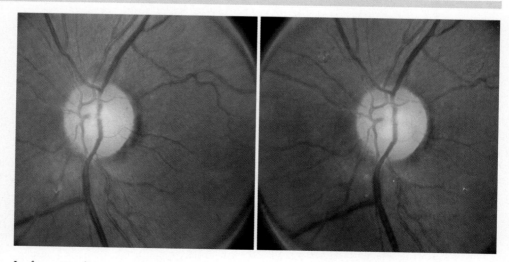

Left optic disc appearance in a patient with a history of methanol ingestion.
In this mild case, the disc has a vertically oriented, deep, oval cup with a
somewhat pale and sloped temporal neural rim. Automated perimetry
showed a small inferior paracentral visual field defect.

Compressive lesions of the optic nerve or chiasm.   **Fig. 19-15**

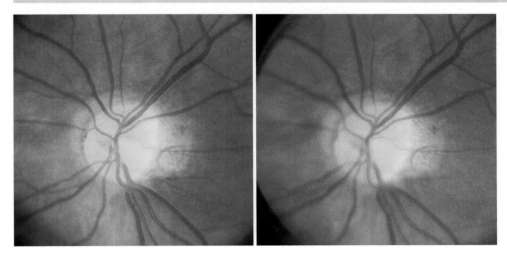

Fig. 19-15A

Left optic disc in a patient with an orbital apex meningioma and elevated intraocular pressure. The left optic cup was slightly larger than the right optic cup, and there was temporally positioned peripapillary atrophy in both eyes. The predominant finding, however, is pallor of the optic nerve tissue in this disc.

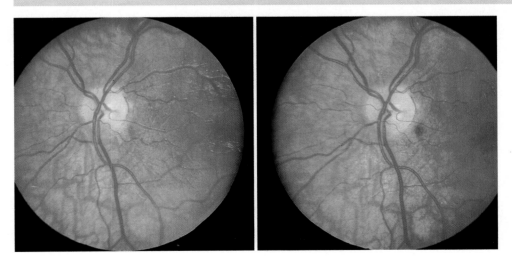

Fig. 19-15B

Pallor of left optic disc in a patient with pinealoma.

Fig. 19-16

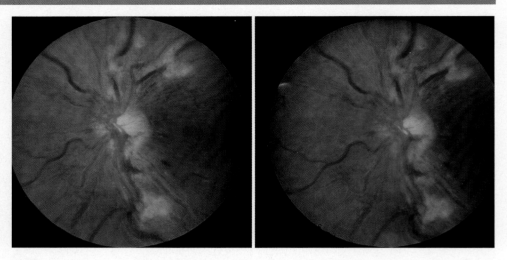

Left optic disc showing acute phase of ischemic optic neuropathy. There is disc edema, hemorrhages of the nerve fiber layer, and cotton-wool spots.

Fig. 19-17

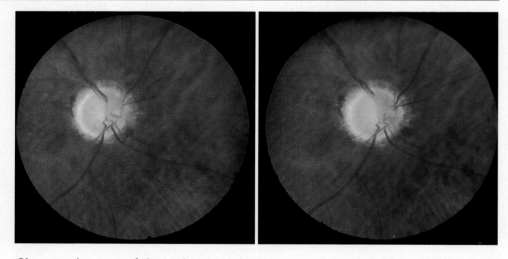

Chronic changes of the right optic disc in a patient with a history of ischemic optic neuropathy. There is pallor of the remaining neural rim, best appreciated inferonasally. There also is cupping of the optic nerve.

INDEX

E

F

G

Sclera
  examination of, 4
  iris melanoma and, 97
  removal of, 9
Scleral melanocytosis, 127
Scleral ring
  of Elschnig, 152, 156
  peripapillary, 152
Scleral spur, 6, 24
  ciliary body tear and, 69
  congenital glaucoma and, 115
  iris process and, 8
  posterior embryotoxon and, 120
  torn tissue and, 68
  trauma to, 62
Sclerostomy, 93
Scotoma
  Bjerrum, 172, 198
  cecocentral, 223
Segmentation of pigmentation, 14
Senile sclerotic disc, 182
Septum pellucidum, 220
Shaffer grade IV angle, 6
Situs inversus, 220
Slit-lamp examination, 4
Slit-lamp gonioscopy, 8
Slit-lamp photography, hyphema, 64
Sphincter, iris atrophy and, 20
Spindle, Krukenberg, 45
Staphylomatous ectasia, 220
Stellate configuration, 11
Stereo fundus photography, 154
Stereo scanning electro micrography, Cogan-Reese
    syndrome, 91
Steroid therapy, uveitis and, 52
Steroid-induced glaucoma, 200
Stoma, 6
Stretch hole, 92
Stroma
  iris, loss of, 120
  removal, 22
Sturge-Weber disease, 126
Suprachoroidal effusion, 146
Surgery, filtration, see Filtration surgery
Swan syndrome, 109
Synechia
  anterior, 29
  irido-corneal-endothelial syndrome and, 87
  iris retraction syndrome and, 136
  peripheral anterior, 90, 91
    essential iris atrophy and, 92

Synechia formation, 55
  abnormal Descemet's membrane and, 86
  inflammatory, 58
  iris bombé and, 59
  traumatic, 66
Synechial angle-closure glaucoma, 93
Synechial closure, 25
  neovascular glaucoma and, 108
Synechial scarring, to trabecular meshwork, 69
Syphilis, optic nerve atrophy and, 224

T

Tilted disc syndrome, 219, 220, 234
Tissue tearing, trauma and, 62
Tonicity, recessive optic atrophy and, 221
Toxic optic neuropathy, 222-2234, 240
Toxicity
  ethambutol, 240
  methanol, 240
Trabecular meshwork, 6
  acute angle-closure glaucoma and, 21
  after traumatic damage, 72
  amelanotic melanoma and, 99
  anterior, 23
  chamber-deepening procedure and, 26
  chronic scarring of, 52
  congenital glaucoma and, 115
  endothelial cells of, 6
  exfoliation glaucoma and, 34
  hemorrhage within, 62
  inflammation of, 55
  inflammatory obscuration of, 81
  keratic precipitates and, 54, 56
  neovascular glaucoma and, 104
  neovascularization of, 108
  obstruction by liquefied material, 78
  outflow channels and, 14
  peripheral iris and, 18
  pigment balls on, 67
  pigmentary glaucoma and, 44
  pigmentation in, 44, 48
  solitary iris process and, 7
  synechial scarring, 69
  tearing of, 68, 70
  trauma to, 62
  traumatic hemorrhage within, 70
  tumors and, 96
Transillumination defect, 47